1980

Assessing and Improving Health Care Outcomes:

The Health Accounting Approach to Quality Assurance

John W. Williamson, M.D.

Technical Editor
Renate Wilson

Ballinger Publishing Company ● Cambridge, Massachusetts
A Subsidiary of J.B. Lippincott Company

International Standard Book Number: 0-88410-706-X

Library of Congress Catalog Card Number: 78-2367

Printed in the United States of America

Library of Congress Cataloging in Publication Data

Williamson, John W
   Health care outcomes.

   Includes index.
   1. Medical care—Evaluation. 2. Medical care—Quality control. 3. Hospital care—Evaluation. 4. Hospital care—Quality control. I. Wilson, Renate. II. Title.
[DNLM: 1. Quality of health care—Standards. 2. Ambulatory care—Standards. 3. Medical audit. WX153 W731h]
RA394.W55   362.1   78-2367
ISBN 0-88410-706-X

To my wife Marlene
and to our daughters, Lori Lynn and Julie Wynne,
with my love and with deepest appreciation
for your support and patience

Contents

Chapter 5
Managing Quality Assurance Information Needs: A Brief
Introduction to Structured Group Judgment and Problems
of Health Sciences Information   99

Part II
Health Accounting—Description and Results of an Outcome
Based Quality Assurance Strategy   117

Chapter 6
The Origin and Structure of Health Accounting   119

List of Tables

List of Figures

Preface

This book explores concepts and methods of an outcome approach to quality assurance in ambulatory and hospital care. Its purpose and scope are twofold: To demonstrate the feasibility and potential of using outcomes as the basic assessment measures in quality assurance in the health professions, and to illustrate this approach with the early results of assessment studies of patient care in a variety of care settings, using the health accounting approach to the assessment and improvement of care. This approach, which is not dependent on available medical records, was developed and tested by the author in the 1960s and early 1970s and is now being implemented at a growing number of health care facilities.

No quality assurance strategy, however well formulated and carefully developed, will be a universal remedy for all the major and minor ills afflicting the field of health care. But while many of its deficiencies are indeed correctable, most present quality assurance suffers from the restrictions of a narrow group of assessment methods that depend almost entirely on the medical record. Chart reviews and medical audits unavoidably omit much of the information needed for quality assurance. What seems to be needed instead is an approach utilizing a wide range of methods that will permit us to focus on the critical problems of care, regardless of the availability of recorded data documenting isolated health care processes and functions. Important aspects—such as provider and consumer values, interests, and motivations—must be addressed, and these require methods of inquiry rarely amenable to chart abstracting. Also, issues such as health care organization and financing; interpersonal and institutional relationships; the assumption of responsibility for continuing care; and provider skills required for health education, lifestyle counseling, and value clarification may ultimately prove important determinants of adequate health or economic outcomes of care. Both the health care establishment and government appear to have recognized these problems and their implications for the future, but despite growing evidence that present quality assurance, continuing education, and regulatory efforts are insufficient to bring about substantial change, there is continued reliance on concepts and mechanisms that fail to go to the heart of the problem.

This book, therefore, proposes, and documents experience with, a prospective approach centering on the measurement and analysis of health care outcomes. For this strategy to be effective, however, the concepts of outcomes must be clarified and meaningfully related to patient and provider values so as to permit identification of health care benefits and disbenefits and of the potential for cost-effective improvement. The emphasis should be on a broader understanding of the concept of health care outcomes, so as to ensure flexibility in the choice of both assessment and improvement modalities at individual, institutional, and community levels and to permit the quantification and measurement of achievable benefits of health care. On the basis of these criteria for an outcome based quality assurance strategy, practical procedures have been developed for local providers to establish standards for evaluating the outcomes of care. Such standards require explicit group consensus on what benefits of care are achievable in the light of current medical knowledge and on the extent to which such benefits must be realized, within the constraints of local resources, to be acceptable to both providers and consumers.

It is hoped that this focus on the achievable benefits of care may contribute to the development of a workable, outcome based quality assurance approach, as well as to a conceptual framework that will facilitate future developments in the field.

Baltimore, Maryland   John W. Williamson, M.D.
January 1978   Professor of Health Services Administration
                                  and International Health
                                  Johns Hopkins School of Hygiene and
                                  Public Health

Acknowledgments

This book reflects a major aspect of the author's work and thinking over a fifteen-year period, and he is thus in debt to many more than can be acknowledged in this space. However, there are several people without whose help this book would not have been possible, and I wish to acknowledge their contributions specifically and with gratitude.

I thank Kerr L. White for the opportunity to continue and expand my involvement in the field of quality assurance and health services research; much of the work reflected in this book was done during his chairmanship of the Department of Health Care Organization at The Johns Hopkins School of Hygiene and Public Health. He not only contributed to the evolution of my thinking on the issues discussed in this book, but provided invaluable organizational support as well, including arrangements for financial support that made it possible to complete this work.

I also wish to acknowledge the contributions of many esteemed colleagues, above all those of Paul J. Sanazaro and George E. Miller, who encouraged me in pursuing the research that was to lead to the development of health accounting. My work at the University of Illinois owes much to their support. I am most grateful as well to Evert Reerink, Paul Batalden, Peter Goldschmidt, Walter McClure, Richard Jeffries, Isidore Altman, and Evelyn Flook for their time in reading several drafts of this book and for their valuable suggestions.

I am especially grateful to Renate Wilson, the technical editor of this volume, for her substantive contributions in rewriting and restructuring a lengthy early manuscript and to Susan Dadakis Horn for her reanalysis of all project data and for providing the statistical framework for reporting their significance and validity.

My thinking on an outcome approach to quality assurance has benefited substantially from the ideas and suggestions of a remarkable group of graduate students with whom I have been directly associated over the years, among them Michael J. Goran, Clement Brown, Joseph Gonnella, Dale Schumacher, John Mitchell, Sidney Kreider, Robert Brook, Kathleen Morton, Robert Dershewitz, David Kern, Dennis Bertram, Peggy Brooks-Bertram, and Richard Gross. Their contributions to the first ten years of health accounting (reported in Part II of this book) and their share in the subsequent development of the concepts underlying this approach continue to be a source of much personal satisfaction and appreciation.

I wish to take this occasion to acknowledge a special debt of gratitude to the American Group Practice Association (formerly the Association of American Medical Clinics) for its cooperation in assuring the participation of many of the clinics and associated hospitals throughout the United States in the 56 health accounting projects reported in this book; to the many health accounting coordinators and health accountants who conducted these studies; and above all to Martin Berdit, the original project director, on whose shoulders fell the difficult task of the simultaneous feasibility testing of 30 health accounting projects in 12 clinics. Filling the roles of research director, education coordinator, and overall program administrator, his competence, untiring effort, and enthusiasm made it possible to demonstrate that health accounting is feasible and replicable. Thanks are due also to many members of The Johns Hopkins University project staff for their efforts in implementing the research and development work reported in these pages, above all to Harriet Braswell, Mark Epstein, John Heimberger, and Susan Lohmeyer. Finally, special thanks are due to Bernice Culp for her patience and skill in typing the manuscript and to William Harris and Judith Flagle for their help with programming and data compilation.

The support of the following organizations is gratefully recognized: The Commonwealth Fund provided financial support to the Office of Medical Education Research of the University of Illinois, under whose auspices health accounting was initiated, and more recently, a Grant-in-Aid for preparing and writing this book. Development of health accounting was supported by the National Regional Medical Programs under Contract PH-43-68-948, subsequently funded through the National Center for Health Services Research, formerly in the Health Resources Administration of the Department of Health, Education, and Welfare, and more recently, by Grant

HS-01590, Grant HS00110, and Grant HS0012 from the National Center for Health Services Research. Generous support was also provided by the Milbank Memorial Fund through a Faculty Fellowship which supported much of the developmental work of the health accounting project and the writing of an early draft of this book.

❋ *Part I*

Basing Quality Assurance
on the Outcomes of Care:
Conceptual Considerations

✳ *Chapter 1*

The Potential for Improvement in Quality Assurance and Health Care

There are few who would question the urgent need for quality assurance in the provision of health care in the United States. Serious concern has been caused by the rising costs of care and the lack of corresponding health improvement in the population. A number of writers have suggested that a substantial portion of present health care expenditures and services might in fact be doing damage to the nation's health. Such commentaries range from the benign criticism of Leon R. Kass, professor of neurology and philosophy at Georgetown University, who stated that "people both in and out of medicine have begun to wonder out loud whether and to what extent medicine is doing good . . ." (Kass, 1975), to the harsh indictment of Ivan Illich, who concluded that "the pain, dysfunction, disability and even anguish which result from technical medical intervention now rival morbidity due to traffic, work and even war-related activities. Only modern malnutrition is clearly ahead" (Illich, 1975: 20-21). The documentation provided by critics such as Illich does not allow us to classify their comments as idle hyperbole or muckraking, and Walter McNerney, president of Blue Cross, has observed that such criticism no longer represents isolated voices but rather a resounding chorus (McNerney, 1976).

Numerous voluntary and regulatory mechanisms have been developed for assessing and improving health care. The national programs of the Professional Standards Review Organizations (PSROs) and the Performance Evaluation Procedure (PEP) adopted by the Joint Commission on Accreditation of Hospitals are meaningful responses to a critical need. Thus, it in no way detracts from these and similar achievements in the field of quality assurance if we ask whether or not such efforts can in fact lead to substantial improvement in the nation's health, a significant reduction in care costs, or both.

That this question requires attention is underscored by a further consideration in the political field. Unless major deficiencies in the current provision of services and the quality of care are corrected, social forces may well take over, as happened in 1973 in the province of Quebec, Canada. There, the passage of Legislative Bill 250 was strongly influenced by the opposition of Quebec physicians to the development of more stringent quality assurance mechanisms. After two-thirds of the medical specialists in the province went on strike, the legislature was forced into action, passing a law that may well set into motion a process of rescinding the privileges of self-regulation for most of the professions in Quebec (Greene, 1976). For when any profession loses sight of social values and becomes inured to public criticism, the danger of increased government regulation is imminent.

Indeed, a recent national population survey and a survey of panels of medical and nonmedical professionals (Goldschmidt, Jillson, and Bordman, 1977) suggest that the medical profession seems to have a somewhat exaggerated perception of the value society has received for the billions of dollars expended on the health industry. The profession would also seem to have ignored much real need in their choice of care priorities and research expenditures. If society is thus beginning to realize that the medical profession is not only stressing the wrong problems, but not doing as well as they might by their own standards, serious conflict lies ahead. Few question that, in the long run, society will have its way. In the evolution of modern quality assurance programs, it would seem crucial that such considerations be acknowledged and made explicit.

It is a working premise of this book that there are several requirements that must be recognized and incorporated into any system of quality assurance if it is ultimately to succeed in terms of substantial improvement of the nation's health or of a significant reduction in care costs. This introduction will outline and discuss these requirements with a view to identifying areas of potential improvement in contemporary quality assurance. It is hoped that this approach will contribute to a framework for the next phase of quality assurance program development in the United States.

REFORMULATING THE CONCEPT
OF HEALTH CARE OUTCOMES

Traditional concepts of health care outcomes, their determinants, and their values may have been adequate when formal methods of evaluating health care were all but unknown and of little concern. However, the present needs of the field have reached a point where such traditional concepts are seriously confining and must be expanded and augmented, a point that will be argued in greater detail in Chapter 2.

The Concept of Health Care Outcomes

While the concept of "outcomes of health care" is probably as old as medicine itself, present use of the term is usually attributed to Donabedian (1966) and his classic paper differentiating between the outcomes, processes, and structures involved in providing medical care. Assessment mechanisms on a national basis were developed first for evaluating structure (facilities, personnel); later, methods for assessing process (what providers do) evolved; and finally, interest and focus on outcomes (results of care provided) developed. This sequence of methodological development is probably attributable to two factors: the relative ease of understanding and quantifying structure and process variables, which facilitated the establishment of assessment standards and measures; and the apparently unshakable belief that structure and process are directly related to health outcomes and therefore provide valid proxy measures of health care benefit.

This may explain the early emphasis on structure, including licensure, accreditation, and certification procedures, for assuring quality of care at state and national levels. While the widespread application of process assessment methods may have been delayed by the complexity of identifying the type, amount, and timing of specific care interventions, growing recognition that certain patient problems required certain interventions that could be enumerated and checked led to national acceptance of process assessment by way of chart review, claims review, and medical audit over a century after acceptance of structure accreditation procedures. Because of the process orientation of traditional medical education, and because of the fact that what providers do in rendering care is apparent and understandable, a crucial weakness of this more recent focus on process was overlooked, namely, the failure to assess explicitly the degree of validity and sufficiency of the evidence linking care structures and processes to outcomes of care in general and to health outcomes in particular. The assumption of the adequacy of such evidence depended upon the acceptance of current medical science information, which few providers questioned.

It was not until an effort was made to develop outcome assessment methods that this problem became recognized. Suddenly, the lack of essential information regarding the natural history of most diseases, and of documentation of treated and untreated prognoses for nearly all health problems, became apparent, as reflected in current interest in the concept of efficacy of care interventions. Erroneously, this information deficiency was defined mainly as a problem of outcome assessment, an association that has in part been responsible for the slow acceptance of outcomes as the focus of assessment. If progress is to be made in developing quality assurance methods, it must be recognized that process and outcome cannot be separated. Identifying deficient outcomes furnishes the most direct assessment focus for isolating deficient processes that require improvement. Improvement of care processes, in turn, is essential if more satisfactory outcomes are to be achieved. In the absence of valid and sufficient information permitting the attribution of specific outcomes to specific processes, therefore, neither process and structure nor outcome assessment systems will prove viable.

Definition of outcome content poses a further problem that may seriously restrict the potential of outcome assessment procedures. Donabedian's original concept seemed to restrict outcomes to health outcomes such as recovery, restoration of function, and survival (Donabedian, 1966). Later, patient satisfaction was included as a positive outcome, and White (1967) stressed negative outcomes in the six Ds: death, disease, disability, discomfort, dissatisfaction, and disruption of productive and social life. As Starfield (1974) pointed out, another problem is the restriction of "outcomes" to end results, inferring final outcomes only and unnecessarily excluding intermediate outcomes. Starfield, however, proceeded to place another restriction on the term, applying it to patient health outcomes only and proposing an outcome profile covering longevity, activity, comfort, satisfaction, disease, achievement, and resilience. She argues that such patient factors as compliance, attitudes, and knowledge or such systems aspects as costs and the availability or accessibility of care should not be included in the concept of outcomes.

In contrast, this book argues that the restriction of outcomes to any specific content, to the exclusion of all other aspects, is a major correctable deficiency of present attempts to develop effective outcome assessment methods. The concept of outcomes in health care is evolving and will continue to evolve. What is necessary now is to recognize that in using the term "outcome," we should not limit its application but emphasize the need to be more specific. In other words, whenever an outcome is assessed, it is essential to state *what* outcome of *what* process, as measured at *what* time. Only then can we test the principles on which assessment measures and quality assurance standards are based, since these principles should be universally applicable, regardless of the specific content measured. The major distinction between current process and outcome assessment methods, for example, has little relationship to what is being measured but rather depends on the assessment design—i.e., the direction of logical inference. One can start by assessing outcomes and, if these are found deficient, apply deductive reasoning to single out determinant processes; or one can measure processes and by induction infer that benefit has been achieved if care interventions are found to be adequate. It is argued here that the deductive approach, working back from deficient outcomes to establish deficient processes, is the most viable approach for most purposes, regardless of assessment content.

The recognition that there are many types of outcomes should not obscure the fact that in most situations, patient health outcomes will be the most important and immediate focus of assessment. However, in other places, at other times, and for other purposes of quality assurance, it may be equally important to measure provider outcomes, such as career satisfaction and attitudes toward patients or health problems, or more general health care results, such as utilization outcomes, economic or political outcomes, and even ethical and legal outcomes.

Determinants of Health Care Outcomes

The second major concept that must be examined relates to the determinants of health care outcomes, and specifically to the evidence linking care processes to outcomes. The latter is the area of health care where practitioners depend most on researchers in the medical sciences and where they are most likely to be seriously disappointed (Williamson, 1977). Establishing evidence of causal associations is a critical aspect of both scientific and practical undertakings. The greater the potential implications of a decision, the more important it is to obtain valid factual information that supports assumptions of the causal relationships involved. For instance, an understanding of the implications of placebo effects is important in analyzing the determinants of health care outcomes (Beecher, 1959). A better recognition of this problem and a more systematic approach to its solution on the part of health care practitioners and quality assurance investigators are essential for the improvement of present health care.

For those doubting this argument, it may be sobering to consider the following example of the attribution of outcomes to specific therapeutic procedures. In the 1950s, internal mammary artery ligation came to be widely used as an efficacious intervention in coronary artery disease, on the assumption that tying off the mammary artery would force greater blood flow through the coronary and other nearby arteries. Health benefits attributed to this procedure included a dramatic increase in exercise tolerance and relief from anginal pain. However, a randomized clinical trial conducted in 1958 to provide evidence of causal relationships between reported health outcomes and mammary artery ligation showed that both the experimental group undergoing the procedure and a control group receiving an operation in which the mammary artery was exposed but not ligated experienced the same health benefits in terms of symptom relief and increased exercise tolerance. This surgical procedure has since been all but discontinued (Cobb et al., 1958; Neuhauser and Johnson, 1974).

This example is one of many illustrating the necessity of systematically and carefully examining the evidence relating health care outcomes to processes. Most medical practice is based on unquestioned assumptions of the validity of associations between diagnostic and therapeutic results and necessary and adequate care processes. A crucial and immediate task of quality assurance is to question these assumptions and to seek more substantial and systematic evidence of the nature of the link between health care process and outcomes.

The Value of Health Care Outcomes
Apart from defining specific health care outcomes and establishing reasonable evidence linking an outcome to a care process, quality assurance requires documentation of its value to the patient or to a larger social group such as the family, community, or nation. The first aspect that must be recognized here is that the value of a given health care outcome is a relative and not an absolute attribute. It may be perceived differently among individuals, or between individuals and larger social groups, quite apart from the fact that it may well change over time. Prevention of pregnancy, for example, may be considered beneficial by the individual or family, but harmful by society, or vice versa. Vasectomy or tubal ligation as contraceptive measures might be valuable at one point in a patient's life and detrimental later when circumstances have changed, as in a subsequent marriage where children are desired.

A second aspect is that the value of any health care outcome represents the sum of three classes of values attributable to any effect:

- Positive (helpful or desired),
- Negative (harmful or undesired),
- Neutral (neither helpful nor harmful).

Rarely will all the effects of a given care intervention fall entirely into one of these classes. Even care producing neither benefit nor damage to health may be completely unnecessary and thus have negative economic value. In other words, for most outcomes, positive, negative, and neutral effects must be considered and weighted, at least in a crude fashion, to determine which value predominates. Experience has shown that quality assurance may be more successful in reducing negative effects of health care than in augmenting its positive effects. That is to say, attempting to obtain the unrealized positive value of health care by correcting errors of omission may offer less immediate promise than the correction of negative effects caused by errors of commission, such as unnecessary medication or surgery, invalid or misleading laboratory test results, and deficient health education, which produce at least economic ill effects for the health care system and perhaps considerable individual anxiety and risk, if not health damage.

The major usefulness of the concepts of health care outcomes discussed here lies in their applicability to the task of formulating a framework for assessing and improving the benefits of current health care. They can also afford a better understanding of the classic evaluation indicators of efficacy, effectiveness, and efficiency, which may well provide the foundation for a more successful approach to developing future quality assurance systems. Here, it may be helpful to consider the evolution of the meaning and use of these indicators in a historical context.

Prior to 1900, writings related to what is now termed efficacy were indexed under the term "certainty in medicine." For example, an article by Bartlett (1848) described the prototype of a clinical trial, supporting the value of leeching for pneumonia. He concluded that although the evidence did not support the assumption of a causal relationship between the use of leeches and a decrease in pneumonia mortality (just as many treated as untreated patients having died at the same stage of disease), the evidence did support a tentative conclusion that leeching was related to reduced symptoms in patients so treated, an outcome not achieved in the untreated groups. In the early 1900s, the term "efficiency" was used to indicate the relative value of medical care to patient outcomes. Codman's famous treatise on hospital efficiency (Codman, 1914) illustrates the use of this word to combine what are presently termed "efficiency" and "effectiveness." In his book on assessing the efficiency of medical care, Querido (1963) explored the concept of efficacy and effectiveness as combined in the term efficiency, and Cochrane (1972) finally popularized the separation of the concepts of effectiveness and efficiency. However, Cochrane's use of the term "effectiveness" still included two concepts: the inherent value of an intervention under ideal conditions (efficacy) and the extent of its potential value as realized in present practice (effectiveness). White made this distinction in a World Health Organization Technical Report (WHO, 1971), where the following definitions were proposed:

- Efficacy: The benefit or utility to the individual of the service, treatment, regimen, drug, preventive, or control measure advocated or applied.
- Effectiveness: The effect of the activity and the end results, outcomes, or benefits for the population achieved in relation to the stated objectives.
- Efficiency: The effects or end results achieved in relation to the effort expended in terms of money, resources, and time.

While a helpful clarification of concepts, the WHO definitions still fail to make an important functional distinction relating to the level and the circumstances where benefits of care are demonstrated. Thus, efficacy should indicate the maximum feasible benefit of an intervention for individual patients or patient populations under ideal conditions of care, such as in a scientific laboratory or clinical trial, while effectiveness should relate to the degree to which both individuals and populations can be shown to have benefited from efficacious interventions in normal or usual conditions of clinical practice. For the purposes of quality assurance application, the following operational definitions are suggested:

- Efficacy: The extent to which a health care intervention can be shown to be beneficial under optimal conditions of care.
- Effectiveness: The extent to which benefits achievable under optimal conditions of care are actually achieved in clinical practice.
- Efficiency: The proportion of total cost (e.g., money, scarce resources, and time) that can be related to actual benefits achieved.

The estimation of health care benefit and of its correlate, achievable benefit not achieved, will be discussed in Chapter 3.

INCREASING AWARENESS OF THE
EVOLVING CONTENT OF
HEALTH CARE

A second major dimension for effecting improvement in present quality assurance systems is the expansion of both their assessment and their improvement activity beyond the traditional boundaries of medical care. Practitioners are increasingly hampered by their traditional orientation to organic medical disease and its associated physical and chemical cures. Failure to recognize the organizational and economic determinants of good health care could prove equally confining. At present, too much of our scarce resources and of professional effort go into managing late stage disease, where the least benefit can be achieved—to the neglect of preventive measures and health education, where much more might be accomplished.

In contrast, the development of methods such as health hazard appraisal and of the concepts of prospective medicine (Robbins and Hall, 1970) have contributed to health care approaches emphasizing risk management and preventive medicine. On a national level, Lalonde (1974) has shown that we must redirect our attention to the problems of humans, ages one through seventy, to obtain a more meaningful idea of health care priorities. He demonstrates the power of considering life years as opposed to crude mortality or morbidity statistics: a patient dying at age 30 represents a loss of 40 life years, as opposed to someone dying at 69, who represents only one life year lost. Thus considered, the leading causes of life years lost are the following:

Motor vehicle accidents
Ischemic heart disease
All other accidents
Lung cancer
Bronchitis, emphysema, and asthma
Suicide
Cirrhosis of the liver

Note that each of these conditions is in some way related to lifestyles and is amenable to effective preventive measures. Furthermore, life-threatening conditions do not make up the bulk of medical practice in the United States, nor, very likely, in Canada. Data from the National Ambulatory Medical Care Survey of Office Practice in the United States (National Center for Health Statistics, 1975), which randomly sampled 645 million office visits for 1973-1974,

Table 1.1   Leading ten presenting complaints and diagnoses, May 1973–
April 1974

As percent of 645 million total US office visits			
Complaints	*Percent*	*Diagnoses*	*Percent*
Nonsymptomatic	36.5[a]	Well patient (Examination without sickness)[b]	17.1
Leg pain/injury	4.0	Acute upper respiratory infections[c]	6.2
Sore throat	3.2	Hypertension	3.5
Headache/dizziness	3.1	Neurosis	2.6
Arm pain/injury	2.9	Chronic ischemic heart disease	2.4
Back pain/injury	2.9	Hayfever	1.9
Cough	2.8	Otitis media	1.6
Abdominal pain	2.5	Obesity	1.6
Cold/flu	2.4	Eczema	1.4
Fatigue	1.8	Refractive errors	1.4
Total	62.1	Total	39.7

Source: National Center for Health Statistics, 1975.

[a]"Nonsymptomatic visits according to patient purposes," NAMCS symptom code categories 900, include 18.5 percent as "nonsymptomatic problems (Codes 900–979), which are predominantly well patient examinations, and 18 percent as "other problems" (Codes 980–999) which are mainly progress visits.

[b]ICDA Code Y00–Y13.

[c]Aggregates "acute upper respiratory infection, site unspecified," "acute pharyngitis," and "acute tonsillitis."

indicate that the ten leading patient complaints, which accounted for 62 percent of the visits, and the ten leading diagnoses, which accounted for 39 percent (see Table 1.1), involve problems that the physician judges to be not or only slightly serious and that often are self-limited.

Any viable quality assurance system must cope with these problems in terms of both assessment focus and improvement potential, so that the practice of medicine and health care can be reassessed in light of the question where the profession might profitably attempt change. By broadening our horizons to include what in fact can be changed, as opposed to merely doing better that which we have traditionally accepted as our responsibility, considerable improvement should become possible. The evidence is becoming rather clear that our present, narrow view of traditional medicine offers only limited scope for significant population health improvement, let alone cost reduction.

Chapter 4 of this book provides a brief overview of those characteristics of patients, health problems, and providers that might be helpful in identifying useful quality assurance topics with a view to health improvement for specific populations. Experience has shown that such considerations are extremely important to the success of quality assurance. For while there are some problems that occur in most health care facilities (e.g., relating to detection and control of hypertension), many if not most topics suitable for assessment and improvement are specific to particular local characteristics of patients, their health problems, and their medical coping abilities; of providers, their specific practice interests, and their experience; and of local facilities and resources. In a recent study of 320 topics nominated for quality assurance study by eight multispecialty clinics throughout this nation, more than 70 percent appeared to be related to only one clinic each and an additional 10 percent to two clinics (Williamson et al., 1978).

Therefore, specific local factors are of as much practical importance as the characteristics of health problems in determining topics for assessment study and for developing reasonable outcome standards in a given practice context. If such a redefinition of the content of health care has merit, a more functional frame of reference might be achieved within which to reconsider the entire field of quality assurance and its most meaningful application to contemporary health care in local practice settings.

DEVELOPING ADEQUATE STRATEGIES FOR MEETING HEALTH SCIENCE INFORMATION NEEDS

Appropriate management of information needs and related decision processes in contemporary quality assurance is a complex and difficult issue. It is usually neglected, probably because of its very complexity and the difficulties encountered in even the attempt to outline and define it; however, it is of crucial importance for the development of practical assessment and improvement strategies. Both more specific scientific and technical information and a widening of the entire information base are required so as to provide more effective strategies for information management and decision making under conditions of uncertainty and rapid technological change. While these requirements can be stated, our ability to cope with them is insufficiently and unevenly developed. Nonetheless, five distinct but interrelated data categories can be outlined that are essential for quality assurance and continuing education purposes:

- *Magnitude and cause of contemporary health problems faced by society*, including their epidemiology and natural history, and

associated functional impairment and disability by etiological categories;
- *Societal values indicating priorities for coping with these problems,* including a delineation of society's perception of the quality of life as related to those impairments that most jeopardize that quality—and for the reduction or elimination of which society is most willing to expend resources;
- *Achievable benefits from health care,* including evidence of the diagnostic validity and therapeutic efficacy of health care interventions in reducing or eliminating such impairments, and information on the availability of the necessary resources;
- *Achievable benefits not being achieved,* including estimates of the effectiveness and efficiency of present health care arrangements in achieving those benefits judged possible of accomplishment within the constraints of available resources;
- *Improvement potential,* including demonstrated means for effecting behavioral and organizational change in those areas where achievable benefits are not being achieved.

The first category of information relates to epidemiology and health status. Information is needed in regard to functional impairments and disability, categorized by etiological classes so as to enable the setting of priorities based on (1) the amount of population impairment involved and (2) demonstrated achievable benefits from current health care management. Recent versions of the International Classification of Diseases Adapted (ICDA) reflected the fact that for most health problems, definitive etiological entities cannot be readily specified. Only four of seventeen categories related to etiology (infective and parasitic disease; neoplasms; congenital abnormalities; and injuries and adverse effects), while most of the remaining categories have been classified according to manifestations of health problems related to anatomical locations and physiological functions (e.g., diseases of the respiratory system, mental disorders, or delivery and complications of pregnancy). The ninth revision of the ICDA will attempt to make these distinctions more clearly and further develop and improve this schema (White, 1978). Future classifications should provide a nosology in terms of correctable determinants of functional impairment. Harmful lifestyle and self-imposed risks (smoking, drinking and driving, inactivity, overeating) may well be major categories on such an axis. At present, such etiological information can only be approximated; it is usually implicit, and its assumptions frequently go unquestioned.

Furthermore, a broad range of health problems must be defined in terms of health status, so as to indicate the amount of functional disability produced in any specified population over time. This should include both length and quality of life. The author has suggested one method of quantifying such disability by measuring the number of population life years that fall into six categories of dysfunction (Williamson, Alexander, and Miller, 1968; Berdit and Williamson, 1973, augmented by Gross, 1977). Direct measures of the quality of life do not exist at the present time, although health status, or its correlate, disability over time, can be approximated in terms of the parameters measured by the National Center for Health Statistics: life years, institutional days, activity limitation days, presence of acute or chronic illness, bed disability days, and days lost from work due to illness.

The second and closely related major category of information essential to health care and quality assurance relates to societal values. Very little is known about which impairments matter most to society, especially in terms of the type and quantity of resources that should be provided to cope with them. Many might prefer a shorter life with greater independence of living to a longer life in a more dependent state. It is a questionable practice, therefore, to assign priorities to health problems on the basis of raw mortality or morbidity data alone, as is often done at present. Not only do we lack data on social values and their relation to resource allocation problems, but there seems to be very little methodological research that would facilitate the acquisition of such data. For example, an interval health scale that would permit adding restricted activity years to symptom or dependent years requires a set of weights reflecting societal values with regard to different levels of impairment. Some investigators (Bush, Fanshel, and Chen, 1972; Berg, 1973) have explored methods that would permit the development of such weights. Again, it is recognized that at this stage, scales can only reflect negative health in terms of functional impairment and disability or their absence. The next stage might include positive health in terms of higher levels of well-being (Ardell, 1976).

The main point in this regard is to emphasize that this type of information is implicit in most health care decisions made at present. By making such expressions of values explicit and more accurate reflections of the values of the populations concerned, including the consumers and providers of health care, and of society in general, more meaningful quality assurance priorities as well as assessment standards can be developed.

The third category of essential information refers to data regarding achievable benefits of health care. It encompasses the base of scientific information regarding causal relationships between care processes and outcomes, especially health outcomes. Documented evidence of the benefits and disbenefits of health care interventions is the most sorely needed and technically the most difficult to obtain. Data regarding available community health care resources are equally necessary for establishing what benefits are achievable for any specified population. Effective and efficient use of present medical capability depends upon the accessibility of human resources and the availability of facilities and financial resources in any given community. Both types of information are needed to determine achievable benefits of health care for specific populations.

The fourth major information category relates to achievable benefits *not* achieved by present care. This category subsumes the other categories mentioned thus far; it requires data on the effectiveness of care in terms of the proportion of achievable health benefits currently not being realized due to errors of both omission and commission, as well as data on the efficiency of care that would indicate the proportion of current health care expenditures spent on harmful or merely useless interventions. The Professional Standards Review Organizations have a specific mandate to obtain data regarding care provided to Medicare, Medicaid, and Title V Maternal and Child Health recipients. Though this development is a starting point, it is restricted in scope, in terms both of the proportion of the national population to which it applies and of the type of health problems concerned. Also, as pointed out before, reliance on medical chart data for the identification of care deficiencies may well hamper efforts to assess and improve overall population health status.

The fifth and final category of essential information concerns knowledge regarding both the theory and practice of effecting behavioral and organizational change. This information is vital for planning improvement. One of the more depressing findings of current quality assurance activity has been the lack of interest in achieving improvement of serious deficiencies. Individual providers are often prone to disregard such problems or to blame them on others and thereby avoid personal involvement in attempts to solve them. A growing body of literature, as reflected in recent reports of the Institute of Medicine of the National Academy of Sciences (1976) and the Health Services Administration's Office of Planning, Evaluation and Legislation (1977), attests to the controversy over the relative ineffectiveness of traditional quality assessment and continuing education mechanisms in identifying problems and achieving improvement. More hopeful, but perhaps equally controversial, is the literature regarding health education of consumers and patients. The well known difficulties in obtaining improved compliance by patients, especially in regard to changes required in lifestyle, attest to the problems in this area.

As difficult as achieving change in individual behavior is the problem of change in organizational behavior. Many problems, such as the motivational effects of payment mechanisms (e.g., in fee for service versus prepaid practice), presuppose changes of the system of care as opposed to the behavior of individual patients or providers. A small but growing body of theory regarding effective methods for dealing with these issues does exist, but it often goes unrecognized. Much that is known is not operational, and that which is operational often does not have an adequate theoretical substructure to qualify as much more than a fad. The recent field of "organization development" (Beckhard, 1969) may lie somewhere in between, depending upon whom one talks to. In any event, this body of information is vital to future efforts at improvement, whether of specific areas of care or of the entire system.

The above five categories of scientific and technical information are essential to modern health care and quality assurance activities, and most policy and decisions undoubtedly stem from implicit, if untested, assumptions regarding the validity of such information. Future improvement will therefore depend on our recognition of these information needs, on the development of new data bases, and on a more adequate interpretation and extrapolation of such data as presently exist. In addition, we must develop skills that permit us to make present assumptions explicit for the purposes of decision making and policy formulation. For if we narrow this discussion of basic information needs to the available literature, we encounter three serious limitations that must be both recognized and managed for the purposes of quality assurance (Williamson, 1977). The first is the problem of relevance, in that much current biomedical information is probably irrelevant to the immediate information needs outlined above; the second problem relates to the validity of that information that is relevant, much of it being either invalid or scientifically unsupported (Karch and Lasagna, 1975; Feinstein, 1974; Gifford and Feinstein, 1969; Schor and Karten, 1966); and the third and equally serious limitation relates to the lack of accessibility of that which is both relevant and valid, since much if not most information is either physically or conceptually inaccessible to those who require it.

Local practitioners, policy staff, and quality assurance personnel have immediate decisional needs that require strategies for coping with these problems of information relevance, validity, and accessibility. The growing methodology of small group judgment procedures may well provide practical help in this regard. By improving the quality and quantity of judgmental input, these methods, which are described in Chapter 5, may well be instrumental in providing a more meaningful information base for a range of quality assurance activities, from the selection of topics encompassing the greatest potential for health impact or efficient resource utilization to the development of outcome assessment standards and measures and the design of effective improvement strategies when deficiencies are found.

REDUCING DEPENDENCE ON PATIENT CHARTS AND READILY MEASURED PROBLEMS

Throughout the history of attempts to assure quality of health care, emphasis has usually been placed on assessment methods that are simple and utilize readily available data. Much of this has been due to the conceptual problems of assessing care performance and outcomes mentioned previously. Perhaps the most substantial evidence for this argument is the fact that whenever assessment has been undertaken, the major focus was on structure, specifically in personnel licensure and later in facility accreditation. Licensure procedures date back to the Middle Ages, more specifically to the court of Roger II of Salerno, where the sacred tradition of examining candidates for recall of isolated facts may well have originated (Riesman, 1936). Candidates with the prescribed educational prerequisites who could pass a formal examination were licensed to practice medicine. It was easier to ask questions of prospective practitioners than to test their patient care performance. In the United States, dating from 1760, when the state of New York established government licensure of physicians (Stevens, 1971), this form of quality assurance has continued to the present day.

Equally important in this country has been the voluntary system of certification of specialty status of physicians by professional medical organizations. Again, the emphasis was and is on pencil and paper tests, sometimes combined with oral examinations, the recall of isolated facts being the major skill required to pass (Levine and McGuire, 1970). Admittedly, use of simulated patient management problems to test problem solving skills has been a significant advance in recent years, but with a view to the practicality of licensing or certifying large numbers of candidates, a narrow range of cognitive skills has provided the major focus.

The recent trend to move beyond sole emphasis on structure to the measurement and assessment of ongoing performance has again made practical considerations such as the availability of data in patient charts and on insurance claim forms a major criterion of present quality assurance systems. Emphasis has been on medical audits, as developed by Lembcke in the early 1950s (Lembcke, 1956). As applied in present PSRO admissions certification and continued stay review and some medical care evaluation studies, if a given proportion of essential care criteria are met, a nonphysician review coordinator can certify the patient's care as being acceptable for payment by the government under Medicare, Medicaid, and Title V requirements, implying that health outcomes will also be acceptable and that unnecessary care has been avoided. Such methods, while a significant advance over previous structure assessment procedures, still must rely on inadequate evidence linking care processes to beneficial outcomes. Practical constraints have resulted in their widespread application, although there is mounting evidence of the counterproductiveness of this trend.

By their very nature, chart review and medical audits often must omit much of the information needed for quality assurance. This is not to deny the value of chart information for certain assessment topics. However, quality assurance activity, to achieve maximum impact, must focus on the critical problems of outcomes, regardless of the availability of current, easily retrieved data documenting isolated instances of health care provision. At present, the practical advantages of chart based systems seem far outweighed by the limited payoff of this approach in terms of health improvement. For example, medical audits may well encourage the provision of even more unnecessary care than is provided at present (Brook, 1974). Nobrega et al. (1977) have furnished convincing evidence of this problem in hypertension management, as well as the more serious finding that process audit may miss over four out of five patients where altered management is indicated by blood pressure (outcome) measures. Nobrega and his co-workers also found that for over three out of four patients flagged by a traditional medical audit, there was no health improvement potential in terms of blood pressure control, since their pressure was already being adequately controlled. Mushlin and Appel (1977) similarly validated chart audit methods as applied in ambulatory clinic practice, finding that audits can miss as many as four out of five patients where outcomes might be improved by altered care, whereas up to three in four cases indicated by chart audit may have little actual potential for health improvement.

In summary, practical considerations have made structure assessment the mainstay of quality assurance in this country for over 200 years, notwithstanding the often recognized limitations in both the scope and validity of such procedures. Despite recent emphasis on more stringent quality assessment methods, practicality is again forcing reliance on process or record based methods that, while a considerable advance over structure assessment, still pose serious problems of both scope and validity. The single most important drawback of the medical audit approach is its narrow focus on problems that can be identified and measured from patient chart or claims form information, thus requiring the use of methods suited to the data, to the neglect of methods that might have greater potential impact in terms of improving patient health.

What is required instead are effective and practicable methods for identifying topics that can lead to an improvement of outcomes, especially those involving patient health. Topics can be selected from several vantage points: specific types of patients, such as culturally deprived or geriatric; specific health problems, whether organic-medical or psychosocial in origin; specific providers, such as physicians, administrators, or the system of practice organization and payment; or any combination thereof. Such a comprehensive approach to the selection of assessment topics will require corresponding flexibility in the development of assessment measures and standards. While present medical information systems may be of help here, important variables will often have to be measured by means of special encounter forms, utilizing prospective assessment designs adapted specifically to the talents and resources of the quality assurance teams as well as to the particular characteristics of the topic. This book has in part been written to demonstrate the feasibility and practicality of such strategies, which are described in Chapters 6-10.

INTEGRATING QUALITY ASSURANCE INTO HEALTH CARE MANAGEMENT FUNCTIONS

Finally, it must be recognized that contemporary quality assurance needs to relate more directly to the day to day practice of medicine; this includes also the internal reward system of most providers, whether individually or organizationally. Today, providers are paid for what they do, not for what they accomplish. There are understandable historical and conceptual reasons for this. However, the very fact that measures of health care actions are not clearly related to health outcomes may explain much of the rising cost, and the often questionable benefits, of contemporary medical practice. In business, profit is a readily understood and easily recognizable goal. By developing financial accounting systems, it is usually possible to maintain an accurate orientation as to where an organization stands in relation to this goal. No one claims to be "too busy" to keep financial records and to assess and improve fiscal status if it results in the reduction of expenditure or an increase of profits or benefits. Providing sound management and fiscal administration is usually a top priority in organizing and running any enterprise.

In the provision of health care, however, there have until now been no feasible mechanisms to define, let alone measure, the benefits of care. The major goal was to provide care—a product that can be defined and measured in terms of utilization variables. However, the results of such care have been automatically assumed to be beneficial in terms of improved health or the quality of life. Consequently, productivity has often been the goal in health care, not effectiveness and efficiency. Most professional self-regulation mechanisms have not only allowed this state of affairs to continue, but have actively encouraged it. Thus, quality assurance functions are now being forced on the profession by external pressures—either assess care, or you will not be paid from Medicare, Medicaid, or Title V funds; either conduct routine quality assurance studies, or have your hospital lose its accreditation. In this frame of reference, quality assurance is not likely to be regarded as of value in itself. With some, it is becoming a game in which organizations learn to satisfy external forces, regardless of how meaningless the function and results may be. Massive chart review mechanisms, by which multiple forms are completed to everyone's satisfaction, often result in little or no impact on such outcomes as the health of the patients or the career satisfaction of the providers and instead may well force overutilization of useless or harmful procedures.

On the other hand, if effective quality assurance is to become an integral part of provider value systems, evidence will have to be established of the cost effectiveness of this approach to health care improvement. It is this author's conviction that if the benefits to patient health of systematic assessment and improvement of care were to be documented more adequately and related to the overall expenditure required to achieve them, both consumer and provider pressures would lead to a more meaningful growth of the field, as discussed in Chapter 11. The ultimate goal is the incorporation of quality assurance functions into the routine management of health care, much as financial accounting and administration are now conducted.

In this book, the participation of 23 health care facilities in the first ten years of health accounting is reported, together with the results of 56 outcome oriented assessment studies. Although the methods underlying this experience were still in the demonstration stage and required development of new skills, procedures, and tools for both research and evaluation purposes, the evidence would seem to support both the feasibility of health accounting as a system and a high level of internal motivation in the implementation of these studies on the part of the providers involved. It is hoped that continued demonstration of the utility, reliability, and validity of this and similar approaches will provide incentives for a more fruitful development of the field as a whole. For if quality assurance in health care remains locked into restrictive, chart centered assessment mechanisms, lack of tangible benefits may well require or provoke more direct external force and regulation. Such a development could be most unfortunate for us all.

REFERENCES

Ardell, D.B. 1976. Meet John Travis, doctor of well-being. *Prevention* 28(4): 62-68.

Bartlett, E. 1848. *An Inquiry into the Degree of Certainty in Medicine and into the Nature and Extent of its Power over Disease.* Philadelphia: Lea and Blanchard.

Beckhard, R. 1969. *Organization Development: Strategies and Models.* Reading, Mass.: Addison-Wesley.

Beecher, H.K. 1959. Measurement of Subjective Responses: Quantitative Effects of Drugs. New York: Oxford University Press.

Berdit, M., and Williamson, J.W. 1973. Function limitation scale for measuring health outcomes. In *Health Status Indexes*, R.L. Berg, ed., pp. 59-65. Chicago: Hospital Research and Education Trust.

Berg, R.L., ed. 1973. *Health Status Indexes.* Proceedings of a conference conducted by Health Services Research, Tucson, Arizona. Chicago: Hospital Research and Education Trust.

Brook, R.H. 1974. *Quality of Care Assessment: A Comparison of Five Methods of Peer Review.* Rockville, Md.: Department of Health, Education and Welfare, Publication No. (HRS) 74-3100.

Bush, J.W.; Fanshel, S.; and Chen, M.M. 1972. Analysis of a tuberculin testing program using a health index. *Socioeconomic Planning Sciences* 6:49-68.

Cobb, C.A., Thomas, G.I., Bruce, R.A., and Merendino, K.A. 1958. Preliminary report of a double blind evaluation of ligation of the internal mammary arteries. *Circulation* 18:704.

Cochrane, A.L. 1972. *Effectiveness and Efficiency: Random Reflections on Health Services.* London: Nuffield Provincial Hospitals Trust.

Codman, E.A. 1914. A study of hospital efficiency as represented by the product. *Trans Amer Gyn Soc* 39:60-100.

Donabedian, A. 1966. Evaluating the quality of medical care. *Milbank Memorial Fund* Q 44(3) pt. 2:166-206.

Feinstein, A.R. 1974. Clinical biostatistics XXV. A survey of the statistical procedures in general medical journals. *Clin Pharmacol Ther* 15:97-107.

Gifford, R.H., and Feinstein, A.R. 1969. A critique of methodology in studies of anticoagulant therapy for acute myocardial infarction. *New Engl J Med* 280:351-57.

Goldschmidt, P.G.; Jillson, I.A.; and Bordman, S. 1977. *A Comprehensive Study of the Ethical, Legal, and Social Implications of Advances in Biomedical and Behavioral Research and Technology.* Summary of the final report for the National Committee for the Protection of Human Rights of Subjects of Biomedical and Behavioral Research. Baltimore: Policy Research.

Greene, R. 1976. *Assuring Quality in Medical Care: The State of the Art.* Cambridge, Mass.: Ballinger.

Gross, R. 1977. Outcome measures of medical care: development and evaluation of a functional status measure for quality assurance. Master of Science thesis, Johns Hopkins University School of Hygiene and Public Health.

Health Services Administration, Office of Planning, Evaluation, and Legislation. 1977. *PSRO: An Evaluation of the Professional Standards Review Organization.* Report Number OPEL 77-12. Rockville, Md.: Department of Health, Education and Welfare.

Illich, I. 1975. *Medical Nemesis: The Expropriation of Health.* London: Calder and Boyars.

Institute of Medicine. 1976. *Assessing Quality in Health Care: An Evaluation.* Washington: National Academy of Sciences.

Karch, F.E., and Lasagna, L. 1975. Adverse drug reactions—A critical review. *JAMA* 234:1236-41.

Kass, L.R. 1975. Regarding the end of medicine. *Public Interest* 40 (Summer): 11-42.

Lalonde, M. 1974. *A New Perspective on the Health of Canadians.* Ottawa: Government of Canada.

Lembcke, P.A. 1956. Medical auditing by scientific methods—Illustrated by major female pelvic surgery. *JAMA* 162:646-55.

Levine, H.G., and McGuire, C.H. 1970. The use of role playing to evaluate effective skills in medicine. *J Med Ed* 45:700-05.

McNerney, W.J. 1976. The Quandary of Quality Assessment. Second J. Douglas Colman Lecture at the Johns Hopkins University School of Hygiene and Public Health, January 28, 1976.

Mushlin, A.I., and Appel, F.A. 1977. Final Report of the Johns Hopkins University Experimental Medical Care Review Organization (EMCRO) Project at the Columbia Medical Plan. Public Health Service Grant No. HS01310 (processed).

National Center for Health Statistics. 1975. *The Ambulatory Medical Care Survey—1973 Summary.* United States, May 1973-April 1974. Vital and Health Statistics, Series 13, No. 21. Rockville, Md: Department of Health, Education and Welfare, Publication No. (HRS) 76-1772.

Neuhauser, D., and Johnson, E. 1974. Managerial response to new health care technology: coronary artery bypass surgery. In *The Management of Health Care,* Abernathy, W.J., Sheldon, A., and Prahalad, C.K., eds, pp. 205-13. Cambridge, Mass.: Ballinger.

Nobrega, F.I.; Morrow, J.W.; Smoldt, R.K.; and Offord, K.P. 1977. Quality assessment in hypertension: analysis of process and outcome methods. *New Engl J Med* 296:145-48.

Querido, A. 1963. *The Efficiency of Medical Care.* Leiden: Stenfert Kroese.

Riesman, P. 1936. *The Story of Medicine in the Middle Ages.* New York: Hoeber.

Robbins, L.C.; and Hall, J.H. 1970. *How to Practice Prospective Medicine.* Indianapolis: Methodist Hospital of Indiana.

Schor, S.; and Karten, I. 1966. Statistical evaluation of medical journal manuscripts. *JAMA* 195:1123-28.

Starfield, B. 1974. Measurement of outcome: A proposed scheme. *Milbank Memorial Fund Q* 52:39-50.

Stevens, R. 1971. *American Medicine and the Public Interest.* New Haven: Yale University Press.

White, K.L. 1967. Improved medical care statistics and the health services system. *Public Health Rep* 82:847-54.

White, K.L. 1978. Personal communication.

Williamson, J.W. 1977. *Improving Medical Practice and Health Care: A Bibliographic Guide to Information Management in Quality Assurance and Continuing Education.* Cambridge, Mass.: Ballinger.

Williamson, J.W.; Alexander, J.; and Miller, G.E. 1968. Priorities in patient care research and continuing medical education. *JAMA* 204:93-8.

Williamson, J.W.; Braswell, H.R.; Horn, S.D.; and Lohmeyer, S. 1978. Priority setting in quality assurance: Reliability of staff judgment in medical institutions. *Med Care* (in press).

World Health Organization. 1971. *Statistical Indicators for the Planning and Evaluation of Public Health Programmes.* Fourteenth Report of the WHO Expert Committee on Health Statistics. WHO Technical Report Series No. 472. Geneva: World Health Organization.

❋ *Chapter 2*

Health Care Outcomes: Their Determinants, Their Value, and Their Importance to Quality Assurance

Few would deny that the outcomes of health care provide the most meaningful assessment measures for quality assurance. However, there is considerable controversy, if not confusion, regarding the definition of outcomes, much of which seems rooted in a narrow conceptualization of this term. The emphasis on health outcomes, for instance, to the exclusion of economic, educational, or social results of care, is both evidence and a continuing source of conceptual misunderstanding, as is the presumed dichotomy between the assessment of process and the assessment of outcomes. The result has been an arbitrary and narrow use of the term that would seem to restrict meaningful application of the basic outcome concept.

To augment the usefulness of this concept for the development of quality assurance, the following prerequisites for measuring outcomes should be established:

- Outcomes of care must be defined in a broad generic sense so as to require specification of *what* outcome of *what* process at *what* time.
- Evidence of causal relations between any given outcome and health care process must be made explicit and subjected to critical analysis regarding its validity.
- The value of health care outcomes must likewise be analyzed, and made explicit, in terms of both their helpful and harmful effects, as perceived by the individual or by a larger social group in a given context of time and circumstances.

25 *91090*

On this basis, it will be possible both to develop the concept of "achievable benefits of care" as applying to those outcomes of positive net value that can be validly attributed to specified health care processes and to define "achievable benefits *not* achieved" (see also Chapter 3) as a point of departure for establishing priorities as to both the content and the degree of effort to be expended on quality assurance.

THEORETICAL CONSIDERATIONS

The Concept of Health Care Outcomes

Health care outcomes should be broadly understood as encompassing any characteristic of patients, health problems, providers, or their interaction in the care process that results from care provided or required, as measured at one point in time. This requires

- Description of all relevant characteristics of patients, health problems, providers, or their interaction in the care process;
- Evidence of causal relationships between such characteristics and any health care provided or required; and
- Specification of the point in time at which such characteristics are perceived and measured.

The first requirement establishes the range of outcomes that can be assessed. Table 2.1 categorizes outcome characteristics by four data classes and indicates that outcomes are not solely confined to patient function or health status. In addition, outcomes can encompass any aspect of the patient and his health problems, of providers, and of their interaction in the care process which permits more specific subsets to be identified for assessment and improvement. Thus, a patient health characteristic to be measured as an outcome might be overall functional impairment (e.g., in personal care or vocational activities), but can equally consist of levels of physical comfort or specific physiological function. Educational outcomes of care might be reduced anxiety as a result of improved medical coping ability, referrals made to health educators, or the patient's understanding and acceptance of his illness as well as the degree of compliance with the prescribed medical regimen. Measurable health problem characteristics in terms of outcomes include not only the status of the individual problem, such as severity of bacterial infection, but also the risk status of selected populations.

Provider outcomes can be measured in terms of the economic rewards of providing care, the satisfaction derived from it, or the

Table 2.1. Examples of measurable health care outcome characteristics by four major data classes

Patient Characteristics[a]	Health Problem Characteristics	Provider Characteristics	Care Interaction Characteristics
Individual	*Individual*	*Individual*	*Individual*
Age/sex	Etiology	Education	Screening
Ethnic background	Topology	Knowledge	Diagnosis
Education	Extent	Skills	History
Health level	Intensity	Attitudes	Physical
Medical coping ability	Stability	Associated personnel	examination
Compliance	Frequency	Physical resources and	Laboratory tests
Knowledge	Stage	facilities	Therapy
Self-care skills	Complexity	Practice organization	Physical
Satisfaction	Natural history	Reimbursement modes	Psychological
Social	Risk factors	Continuing education	Social
Family	Symptoms		Education
Friends	Complaints	*System*	Legal-ethical actions
Community	Abnormal findings	Community resources	Responsibility for care
Occupation	Syndromes	Availability and accessibility of services	Continuity of care
Religion	Diseases	Professional organizations	Utilization
Environmental	*Social and environmental*	Production facilities	Financial
Geography	Analogous to individual health problem characteristics but referring to population health problems, e.g., occupational accidents	Marketing facilities	Time
Climate		Financing systems	Resources
Food supply			*Population*
Water supply			Epidemiological surveys
			Public health services
			Environmental health services
			Production activities
			Marketing activities
			Financing activities
			Legislative activities

[a] Independent of specific health problem manifestations.

knowledge gained that can be applied to other patients, as well as in terms of the effectiveness of provider distribution—e.g., their availability and accessibility. The interaction between the patient, the health problem, and the provider in the care rendered or utilized can provide productive topics for assessment and improvement. The utilization outcome of diagnostic care for a patient might be the aggregate total of laboratory tests ordered or completed or of diagnostic referrals made; the utilization outcome of therapeutic care might be the aggregate total of injections given, surgery performed, or drugs prescribed. Similar characteristics can be defined for groups of patients, health problems, or facilities. For instance, outcome assessment of hospital care could focus on aggregate utilization outcomes such as bed turnover, specific inpatient service rates, or the volume of claims processed.

It should be clear from this definition of outcomes that traditional utilization review studies actually measure outcomes of the health care process. Likewise, the PSRO profile analysis procedure requires the measurement of care interaction outcomes. The range of outcomes that can be assessed is broad; however, this must not obscure the fact that some outcomes may be far more significant than others in any given context. The overriding importance of patient health outcomes should be self-evident. The object here is to show the full spectrum of measurable outcomes and to emphasize that choosing which outcome to measure is one of the basic functions of quality assurance activity, regardless of the system applied. Thus, the basic principles of outcome assessment should apply irrespective of the particular content of the outcome evaluated, whether health status, diagnosis, or therapy, and of whether they are applied at the individual, group, institutional, or population level.

The second requirement, i.e., evidence relating an outcome characteristic to care provided or required, is equally important. The assessed outcome should follow the use of health services in time, and there should be reasonable evidence for its attribution to the care provided. Traditionally, at least at the individual patient management level, antecedent care has been thought of only in terms of direct provider actions such as surgery or writing a prescription, thus limiting the scope of the care process and the factors that could be assessed. Instead, health care should be considered in a much broader context. The recognition of the health problem by the patient or physician, patient self-care based on health education, the physician's management of the problem, and compliance of the patient with that management are all vital aspects of care.

The probability of a causal relationship between health care processes and outcomes may be very high, as in the improvement, after an injection of insulin, of a patient in a diabetic coma. More often, however, such evidence is much less clear-cut. This may be due to the number of factors intervening between a specific care action and the resulting outcome, such as the need to consider placebo effects, as well as to the difficulty of assigning relative weights to such factors or the impossibility of identifying all of them. The best evidence of the effects of medical intervention is that obtained from such research procedures as long-term controlled clinical trials. At present, however, such information exists for only relatively few interventions, and in most situations, medical care is based on implicit assumptions of causality. For the purpose of quality assurance, the validity of these assumptions must be explicitly examined, ideally with a view to determining levels of expert consensus, an aspect discussed more fully in Chapter 3.

The concept of outcomes as developed here also stresses that outcomes are the result of care provided *or* required. The failure to seek or provide needed care can be the cause of a deficient outcome as much as inadequate care; for example, metastatic breast carcinoma because of failure to seek or provide a breast examination.

The third and final requirement, i.e., a specification of the point in time at which the characteristics in Table 2.1 are perceived and measured, is likewise crucial to the function of outcome assessment. The process of health care is a continuum. Throughout a lifespan, care may be required and/or provided at any time, whether in the form of prenatal care, management of acute or chronic health problems during life, management of terminal illness, or even as relating to the care of organs transplanted after the death of the patient himself. Characteristics of any of these aspects of the overall care process can be described at any point on this continuum; they may change radically with the passage of time. Likewise, quality assurance implications of measuring a specific characteristic may change over time. Focus on early detection of breast carcinoma would seem to have far greater assessment benefit than focus on late stage disease, if a choice were required. Determining which characteristic to examine at what stage in order to optimize improvement potential is a major goal of quality assurance planning.

The Continuum of Care—An Infinite Number of Outcomes

The analogy of a motion picture may illustrate the relationship between the care process continuum and a given outcome. What appears on the screen as a dynamic ongoing event represents process.

The content of any single frame of the film represents outcome—in other words, the status of one characteristic as determined by some antecedent process or series of processes. By this analogy, process relates to an infinite series of characteristics, with some, such as patient blood pressure, changing and others, such as patient height, remaining stable during much of the film.

This continuum can be depicted in various ways. It may be expressed as a curve of care activity over time, as in Figure 2.1, or it may be divided into the previously discussed component elements reflecting the patient, the health problem, the provider, or the care interaction among them. Figures 2.2-2.5 show some of these continua as they might apply to a single patient. Figure 2.2 shows, for this patient from birth to age 75, three health status continua for physical impairment in whatever form (Figure 2.2A), overall discomfort (Figure 2.2B), and any impairment of major life activity (Figure 2.2C). Figure 2.3 shows two continua for the health problem experienced by the same person, indicating that asthma symp-

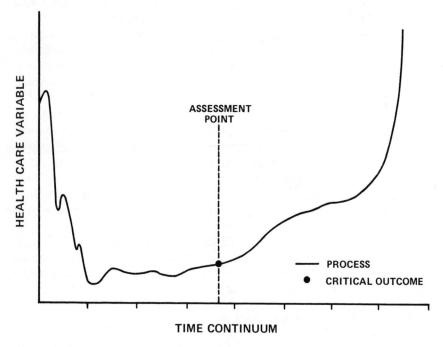

Figure 2.1. The health care process-outcome continuum over time, where a critical outcome judged to be probably deficient is chosen as the assessment point.

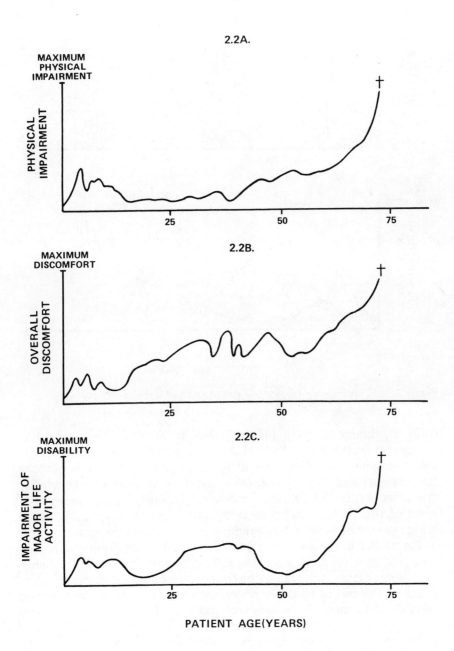

Figure 2.2. Three continua of patient health and functional status over time.

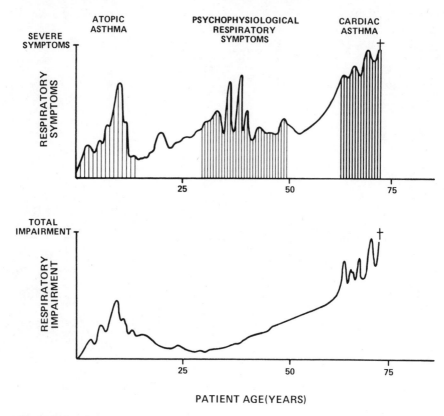

Figure 2.3. Continua for respiratory symptoms and impairment over time.

toms in childhood were probably due to allergy; that respiratory symptoms in the patient's middle years might be of psychophysiological origin, since there was little or no physical cardiorespiratory impairment; and that symptoms in later years were due to cardiac failure as confirmed by other evidence. Obviously, adequate management of this respiratory problem should vary according to the underlying cause, which, as in this example, may change over time.

Figure 2.4 illustrates a provider characteristic, measured as accessibility of care to the same patient. This factor is also seen to change over time. Figure 2.5, which illustrates the care process interaction in terms of the use of health services, indicates an independent though related continuum. Since care was relatively inaccessible in the area where the patient lived, his diagnosis of asthma was never formally reevaluated; after that initial care interaction, treatment was episodic and crisis oriented. Note that utilization of care can be independent

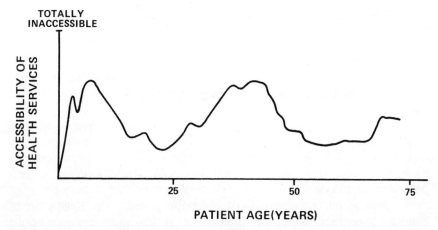

Figure 2.4. Continuum showing accessibility of health services for a patient over time.

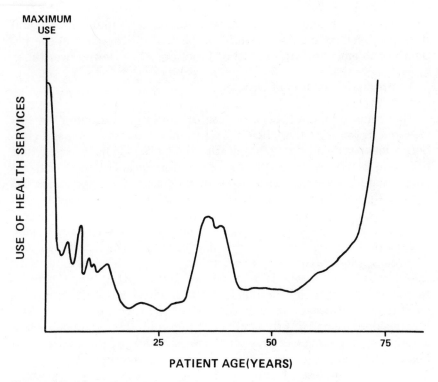

Figure 2.5. Care interaction continuum showing use of health services for a patient over time.

of accessibility of care. When the patient is experiencing serious distress, he will seek medical help, whether from a neighbor, a healer, or the formal health care system (Kohn and White, 1976). Although asthma symptoms and overall discomfort levels remained rather high throughout life, they caused the patient to miss work or to seek care only infrequently during his productive years (see Figures 2.2, 2.3, and 2.5).

For all of these continua, outcomes could be measured at any point in time. The patient's overall level of impairment could be measured at 4 years, or several continua could be combined to yield what might be the most relevant outcome: the degree of impairment of major life activity, especially after any treatment provided. Just as all the elements of care—the patient, the health problem, the provider, and their interaction in the care process—could be combined on one care continuum, specific elements can be combined to form the most useful continuum for a particular assessment focus. The important point here is that the choice of which continuum to assess must be made consciously and with an understanding of the underlying problem etiology, natural history, and status, as well as of the potential impact of health care on the patient's problem, comfort, or level of function, all as viewed over time.

Traditional Concepts of Outcomes and Process

The main distinction between use of the term "outcome" in this view and its traditional application is primarily a matter of specificity. Some investigators, for example Starfield (1974), have urged that this term be confined to patient health outcomes. Others consider it appropriate only as applied to end results or final outcomes. As discussed in Chapter 1, in the context of quality assurance such conventions tend to confine the potential of the outcome concept. Likewise, the term "process" has traditionally been restricted to care actions of the provider, if not the physician. Acceptance of measures of process, such as patient chart information, as synonymous with the care process itself is widespread. Hence, the term "process assessment" is generally applied to the medical audit. It should be clear from the foregoing, however, that care processes should rather be considered part of a dynamic continuum producing specific characteristics, or changes in previous characteristics, of the patient, the health problem, the provider, and their interaction. To actually measure this process of care requires direct observation over time; most surrogate measures of process, obtained at one time (e.g., patient chart entries or insurance claims forms), are actually measures of outcomes of care. The measurement of such outcomes can thus provide only indirect or inferential evidence of process, as opposed to the direct evidence of observation, as by audiovisual means. Medical process audits therefore suffer from a basic problem: they are based on what are in fact outcome measures that only infer medical care process, and if the process in turn is judged adequate, it again can only be used to infer the adequacy of health outcomes.

The first inference may be fairly safe, but it must be scrutinized to establish whether outcomes can indeed be considered valid surrogates of process. For example, if a hematocrit report indicates a certain value at one time, one may or may not be able to accept the laboratory process by which that value was generated. An expert observer might note that the method applied to obtain the hematocrit could not possibly have yielded a valid result. Surgical or psychotherapeutical procedures are other instances where it would be quite hazardous to infer technical competence by looking at the patient chart only. However, most process assessments are done in just this manner; the mere fact that chart evidence is found, and that the care process was recorded, is usually accepted as sufficient evidence that the procedure itself was validly and adequately accomplished.

The second inference is even more tenuous. Inferring the adequacy of health outcomes from evidence that care processes were provided, even assuming each process to have been adequately and validly represented by patient chart data, is only as valid as the available evidence of causal relations between the care process and health outcomes. Again, this may or may not be a safe assumption, and whether traditional concepts of both outcomes and processes can provide a valid basis for quality assurance is open to serious question. What is required instead of inferences is a systematic examination of antecedent processes to establish reasonable evidence of causal associations.

Outcome Determinants

The attribution of outcomes to specific causes must take into consideration multiple extraneous and intervening variables. In determining the origin of many chronic impairments, for instance, numerous factors must be disentangled to identify which medical intervention may be, or may have been, effective. Unfortunately, most interventions generally considered beneficial and traditionally prescribed are not likely to be based either on documented evidence or on formal consensus on whether they are helpful, to whom, to what extent, and under what circumstances. The effects of radical or simple mastectomy on breast cancer, the use of anticoagulants in myocardial infarction, the multiple cough and cold remedies on the market, the benefit of treating adult onset urinary tract infections in preventing chronic renal failure or of low salt diet in preventing essential hypertension, are all essentially unproven. One of the few examples of systematic documentation of such evidence is the Food and Drug Administration's program of expert team analysis of available research data to verify causal links between the use of pharmaceuticals and specific patient health outcomes (National Research Council, 1969). However, the sufficiency of the evidence on which the attribution of outcomes to specific causes is to be based is an essential consideration in quality assurance. If deficient outcomes of care cannot be traced back to correctable care processes, quality assessment is not likely to be worth the effort. What is needed, then, is a careful examination of the nature of this evidence.

The most clear-cut evidence is provided by a manifest link between antecedent care and outcome, i.e., one that can be readily and validly measured or perceived by observation or deduction. A brief history indicating that a diabetic patient had not been taking insulin would provide manifest evidence of the cause of diabetic acidosis. Putting on a pair of properly refracted eyeglasses provides immediate evidence linking the glasses to improved vision. If such manifest evidence is available, there should be little difficulty in achieving agreement as to the probability of the link between causes and outcomes. Here, controlled trials and sophisticated statistical analyses are probably unnecessary.

Establishing the link between therapeutic outcomes and care processes depends upon how well the natural history of a health problem is known. For example, the five year case fatality rate of gastric carcinoma is generally accepted as being higher than 85 percent. If a treatment were to reduce this rate by half, it would have manifest evidence of efficacy at least as valid as the original medical evidence establishing the untreated case fatality rate. If the natural history is unknown or highly variable, however, more rigorously established evidence is required if valid causal inferences are to be made.

For the larger group of medical care interventions where manifest evidence of causal links to outcomes is lacking, carefully designed and controlled research studies are required. A poorly designed study may yield no more than a series of dubious or coincidental associations, if not serious misinformation, as was the case in early clinical studies of internal mammary artery ligation (Neuhauser and Johnson, 1974). For diagnostic interventions, replicated validation studies are required that measure results of the test being studied against an acceptable criterion test—for example, by validation of premorbid electrocardiogram results against autopsy data for the same patients. For therapeutic interventions, replicated, long-term controlled clinical trials will often provide the only acceptable evidence of treatment efficacy. The most promising research efforts in this regard involve complex studies designed so that the providers giving the experimental treatment are independent of those who evaluate the effects of the treatment. Also, the experimental treatment is randomly allocated, so that the group given the test therapy is similar in every possible way to the second group, which is given a similar but inert treatment. Until the end of the study, it is not known which patient received the experimental treatment. Often, the effects to be measured can only be observed over many years of longitudinal study, as in the University Group Diabetes Study, which has been in progress since 1961 (University Group Diabetes Program, 1970; Goldner, Knatterud, and Prout, 1971; Knatterud et al., 1971).

The validity of research evidence thus depends on the sophistication of the research design and the rigor with which it is applied. However, investigations using stringent criteria are limited by the availability of qualified research personnel and funds and of topics satisfying both practical and ethical constraints, not to mention the innumerable technical and practical problems that can seriously limit the validity of the study findings. The need remains incredibly large. In the meantime, most clinical decisions must be based on individual physician assumptions about the sufficiency of the evidence attributing outcome to treatment. Even when valid studies are available, a physician must make inferences from the results of a study in a specific population to his own, often significantly different, practice setting. An example is the Veterans Administration Cooperative Study, which investigated hypertension therapy for a group of 40 to 55-year old hospitalized male military veterans (Veterans Administration Cooperative Study Group, 1972, 1970, 1967). Can those results be applied to a group including 35-year old ambulatory females? Further, can the research conditions under which evidence of efficacy was identified be generalized to the conditions in which actual diagnostic or therapeutic care will be rendered? To the extent to which the conditions differ, the overall validity of causal inferences between the particular intervention and its outcome may be weakened.

Finally, where both manifest evidence or valid research data supporting causal inferences are lacking, the physician must depend upon experiential or judgmental evidence. Though such evidence has the lowest face validity, its importance lies in the fact that it is all that is available to support many, if not most clinical decisions. For the purpose of quality assurance, the validity of such evidence linking care processes to outcomes will depend upon the depth and range of experience of the physician, in conjunction with the method by which judgmental evidence is obtained. Implicit individual judgment probably has the least validity, whereas explicit, structured expert group consensus will generally provide the most valid experiential evidence of causality that can be obtained in the absence of specific research evidence.

Explicit formal group consensus on the sufficiency of evidence of causality, whatever its source, is advocated for quality assurance on the grounds that explicit judgments are better than implicit judgments, that several experts are better than one, and that systematic methods for eliciting judgments are better than haphazard methods (see also Chapter 5). Such methods have been established and formalized as procedures in the Health Benefit Analysis Project (Emlet et al., 1971). An iterative process is applied in which formal group estimates are obtained, discussed in the light of available research or epidemiological data or literature, and revised, if warranted. This approach, which resembles a modified nominal method of eliciting judgments, permits the synthesis and evaluation of original data estimates and is supported by a growing body of evidence (Delbecq, Van de Ven, and Gustafson, 1975; Williamson et al., 1978). Until sufficient research evidence is available for a wider range of health care interventions, experiential evidence will unavoidably predominate, whether developed formally, systematically, and explicitly by group consensus or informally, haphazardly, and implicitly by an individual.

The Value of Health Care Outcomes

Last, to establish a more functional basis for quality assurance, the value of health care outcomes must be determined. Establishing that specific care processes are determinants of specific outcomes does not provide any information regarding the value of the outcome to the individuals or populations involved. In both medical practice and quality assurance, however, this process of valuation must be understood for purposes of decision making. Just as it is essential to obtain evidence linking care processes to outcomes, so it is essential to obtain specific information of a very different sort to determine the value of any given outcome. Whereas data from diagnostic validation studies or controlled clinical trials are needed to support causal inferences, sociological and psychological data are required to establish to whom a given outcome is of value for what purpose and when and under what circumstances. For this, an understanding of the social context and of the value systems of patients, providers, and society is essential.

Again, terms reflecting values have been used in a narrow and restrictive sense, mainly referring to patient health outcomes and usually in relation to the individual patient. In terms of efficacy, for instance, only positive values have been encompassed and related to care interventions as a universal characteristic, often neglecting harmful side effects or risk-to-benefit ratios, particularly for the long term. For example, insulin is considered efficacious for diabetes, although such labeling obscures the fact that the same intervention can be very damaging to the same person with the same disease in a different context (e.g., by giving more insulin to treat insulin shock misdiagnosed as acidosis) or to different individuals with the same problem (e.g., insulin used in insulin independent diabetes).

The value of interventions also varies depending on whether it applies to the individual or the larger social group. Smallpox vaccine applied to those exposed to whatever of this disease is left in the world could be salutary, yet when applied to large populations, more people might die of cowpox caused by the vaccine than would have died from smallpox itself. Likewise, an intervention might have a positive health value to the individual (e.g., artificial prolongation of life in terminal illness), but serious economic consequences for the family or society. Genetic screening or amniocentesis may be of emotional or economic value to the family in preventing birth of seriously malformed children requiring institutional care but be an entirely negative intervention for "right to life" advocates or have serious ethical effects on the wider social group in certain religions. Clearly, the issue involves value conflicts that must at least be made explicit if the benefit (or disbenefit) of any outcome of health care provided or required is to be established.

In determining the value of any health care intervention or its outcome, two major considerations must thus be addressed. The first encompasses, as suggested above, specification of value content—namely, of value to whom, for what purpose, and under what circumstances. The second lies in recognizing that value is an aggregate concept involving the sum of positive, negative, and neutral effects of health care.

The question, "of value to whom," requires specification of whether we are talking about individuals, groups, or populations. This must above all be recognized in considering conflicts between individual rights and social responsibilities. Preventive health behavior (e.g., cessation of smoking) may have an immediate negative value for the person who must suffer withdrawal symptoms, in spite of its long-term positive health value. Consequently, the smoker may prefer to assume the attendant risk, which is his right. The same outcome (cessation of smoking) may be of immediate positive value for nearby nonsmokers, who are thus protected from the discomfort, if not physical risk, of inhaling the smoke from other people's cigarettes and of even greater positive value for society, which otherwise would have to assume the financial costs of the increased risk of morbidity and mortality that smokers inflict on themselves. Such costs are assumed either directly, through higher insurance premiums, or indirectly, in compensation for lowered productivity and lost talent related to the markedly increased chronic respiratory and cardiovascular illness and premature deaths among smokers. With so much current morbidity and mortality due to problems of lifestyle, these value conflicts between individuals and larger social groups are becoming painfully evident.

The second question, "of value for what purpose," has long been recognized—for instance, in pharmaceutical evaluation studies. Health care interventions may have considerable value for highly specific indications, but little or no value when applied for other purposes. Exotic, expensive laboratory procedures may be valued by the physician who wishes to satisfy his personal curiosity, but if the probability of yielding important information in terms of patient management or prognosis is small, they may be of little value to the patient. Likewise, the risk-to-benefit ratio of surgical procedures may have to be weighed carefully and, if possible, in the light of the patient's own value scale. The main consideration here is that the value of an intervention or outcome must be defined and, where possible, quantified in relation to specific purposes. Otherwise the tendency is to overgeneralize and to invalidly attribute value to applications where it is not warranted, an all too common occurrence illustrated by the propagation of vitamins and iron rich tonics.

Finally, the question of time and circumstances must be recognized in establishing the value of health care interventions or outcomes. The application of potent drugs such as digitalis may be valuable at one point in time and damaging when applied to the same patient for the same problem at a different time; cardiopulmonary resuscitation can be highly valuable at one point and worthless if started an hour later. In other words, the value of an intervention is strongly dependent upon the circumstances, which may be highly dependent upon time.

Equally important is the second major consideration, which is based on the concept of "net value" as the sum of the helpful, harmful, and neutral effects of health care at a given level of social organization. All health care interventions, let along aggregate sets of interventions, have multiple effects, each of which may have a different value. Some effects are obvious health advantages (e.g., penicillin may prolong productive life); however, the same intervention can have simultaneous effects that might be disadvantageous (alteration of normal body bacterial flora) or even fatal (if the patient should have an allergic reaction to the penicillin and die). What is important to recognize is that each of these multiple effects can be classified as either helpful, harmful, or neutral—that is, neither helpful nor harmful. Thus, health care benefits must be defined in terms of their aggregate or "net value" for the individual or populations.

In summary, establishing the value of health care outcomes depends upon three root factors, all of which must be made explicit and analyzed. The first involves precise definition of the outcome of health care involved; the second, establishing adequate evidence that the outcome is indeed attributable to health care; and the third, definition of the value of the outcome in the context of the question, of value to whom, for what purpose, and at what time and under what circumstances? The first can be established by consensual definition; the second requires valid scientific evidence; and the third requires value clarification.

APPLICATION OF THE OUTCOME CONCEPT TO QUALITY ASSURANCE

These concepts of medical care outcomes, their determinants, and their value have useful quality assurance implications. The more important ones relate to the task of identifying outcomes whose assessment might have the greatest impact in terms of health improvement or more efficient resource utilization. An analytical approach to identifying such critical outcomes by means of a chain of associated factors is suggested in the following, in conjunction with several considerations that must be borne in mind when identifying outcomes for quality assurance purposes.

Critical Outcomes
Figure 2.6 illustrates a useful method of deducing and diagramming the relationship of health care processes to critical outcomes. For purposes of the discussion, the outcome shown at the far right of the chain of potentially relevant medical and nonmedical factors in Figure 2.6 is both the end point of the chain and the point of de-

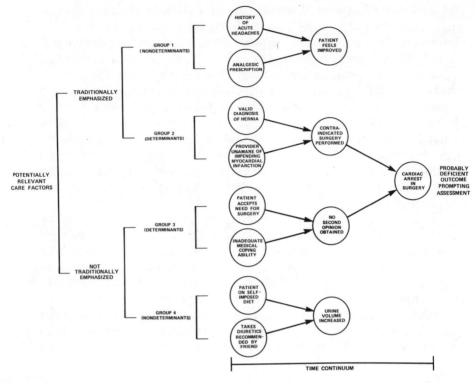

Figure 2.6. Chain of associated factors of potential relevance to outcome prompting asessment.

parture for quality assessment; however, this outcome, as well as all other outcomes depicted, are only points on a continuum encompassing patient, health problem, provider, and care interaction aspects. This chain of associated factors, depicted as a branching logic tree, is a construct that focuses assessment and evaluation on a critical, probably deficient, outcome, together with determinant processes and antecedent outcomes. Each outcome is the result of a hierarchy of preceding processes and outcomes, and the selection of an outcome for assessment should be based on its significance in the chain and on the further requirement that it must represent a measurable result encompassing potential for improvement.

It is a precondition, therefore, that the potential for increased health benefit or more efficient resource utilization is worth the effort required to achieve assessment and improvement, an aspect discussed in greater detail in Chapter 3. It is important to note here that in the chain of associated factors in Figure 2.6, four groups can be identified, two of which would not be considered part of the medical care process by traditional assessment methods. Medical coping ability (an example of Group 3 factors in Figure 2.6) is often as crucial an outcome determinant as are the medical interventions provided (an example of Group 2 factors). Even if such determinants are traditionally considered "nonmedical" factors, they might nonetheless represent valuable topics for quality assurance; for instance, if lack of transportation prevents the followup visit required for a repeat prescription, then this aspect of noncompliance may be an important correctable determinant of an unfavorable outcome of medical care. Conversely, among the groups of associated factors traditionally emphasized in the medical care process, those falling into Group 1 may on closer examination be revealed as irrelevant to the key outcome.

In outcome assessment planning, the establishment of a chain of associated factors is directed backward in time. On the process continuum, an outcome is selected for assessment, and among the network of related factors, the most relevant, measurable, and correctable determinants are specified. To take up our previous analogy, this provides a systematic tool for identifying those points where it might be most meaningful to stop the motion picture projector and examine a single frame—in other words assess a given critical outcome.

Developing a Critical Outcome Chain

The first step in developing a chain of associated factors leading to a critical outcome is the selection of a significant and probably deficient outcome as the starting point for the assessment process. Although several theoretical aspects must be kept in mind, the most important considerations here are the extent to which the outcome of a given health care intervention can be improved and the effort required if quality assurance were undertaken. Thus, outcome selection is basically a cost effectiveness decision, and it involves many assumptions regarding both achievable benefits and the cost of undertaking an assessment and improvement effort. As will be discussed in Chapter 5, this procedure can be facilitated by use of structured group judgment processes for estimating required data that may not be available or existent.

The second step in the analysis consists in determining antecedent outcomes and processes that contributed to the measured deficiency. Since there usually are numerous determining factors that might be shown, it is important to identify those that will be of greatest utility for assessment planning. Thus, only those processes and outcomes should be included that meet the following qualifications:

- They are readily measurable.
- There is acceptable evidence of causal linkage.
- They involve correctable deficiencies.
- There is reasonable evidence that improvement is feasible within the constraints of present resources.

Figures 2.7 and 2.8 illustrate the importance of establishing a chain of specific associated factors in planning assessment of a deficient outcome. When quality assessment measures and standards are developed on the basis of implicit and nonspecific relationships only, as in a chart audit, the result may be similar to that in Figure 2.7. A number of traditionally applied medical care interventions and

	DOCUMENTED IN CHART
HISTORY	
DURATION OF HYPERTENSION	☑
DESCRIPTION OF HEADACHES	☑
PAST HISTORY RENAL, CARDIO-VASCULAR, OR CEREBROVASCU-LAR SYMPTOMS	☑
FAMILY HISTORY OF HYPERTENSION	☑
PRIOR TREATMENT	☑
PHYSICAL EXAMINATION	
SERIAL BLOOD PRESSURE READINGS OVER SEVERAL MONTHS	☑
BLOOD PRESSURE BOTH ARMS	☑
PERIPHERAL PULSES	☑
FUNDUSCOPIC EXAMINATION	☑
EXAMINATION OF HEART, LUNGS, AND ABDOMEN(FOR BRUIT)	☑
LABORATORY	
COMPLETE BLOOD COUNT	☑
URINALYSIS	☑
BLOOD UREA NITROGEN, SERUM POTASSIUM AND VANILMANDELIC ACID IN URINE (24 HOUR SPECIMEN)	☑
ELECTROCARDIOGRAM	☑
ROENTGENOLOGY	
RAPID SEQUENCE IV PYELOGRAM	☑
CHEST X-RAY P-A AND LATERAL	☑

CONCLUSION: ADEQUATE CARE— STROKE NOT PREVENTABLE

Figure 2.7. Hypothetical example of a medical chart audit of care process to infer acceptability of outcome for a forty-two-year old patient who suffered a stroke (criteria as recorded in Payne et al., 1976).

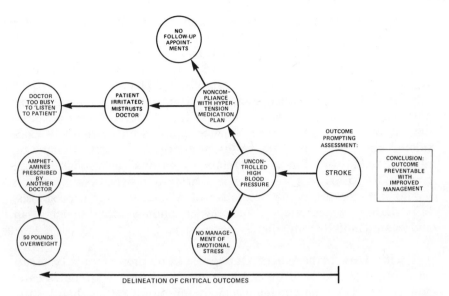

Figure 2.8. Analysis of associated factors for the same patient, directed backward in time to deduce correctable determinants of potentially deficient outcome.

processes might be listed and considered relevant to care, without specifying their causal association. The audit results in this figure would indicate adequate care, leading to the inference that the stroke was not preventable. On the other hand, a deductive approach as depicted in Figure 2.8 indicates that such traditionally emphasized factors make up only one subgroup of factors, all of which may be important. Here, the stroke is considered preventable, as analysis of the specific factors would indicate that the outcome in Figures 2.7 and 2.8 might be attributable to inadequate care. Thus, unacceptable outcomes can be deductively evaluated to test whether they were due to errors of omission or commission in a particular branch of the chain.

Selecting Outcomes for Quality Assurance— Some Practical Considerations

Conclusiveness of Outcomes. An important aspect in the selection of health outcomes for assessment is their conclusiveness, that is, the extent to which the outcome measured predicts an irreversible or stable final result, often termed an "end result." Conclusiveness usually depends upon establishing an optimum interval of time for outcome measurement following therapy. The natural history of a given health problem provides the most meaningful time frame for determining this interval, which can vary widely. A bone fracture may require six to twelve months after treatment before a conclusive or final outcome can be established. The status of a patient recovering from an appendectomy may be provisionally accepted as conclusive within a week, in contrast to the outcome for a cancer patient responding well after a mastectomy, which cannot be considered conclusive for years, as the presence of metastases may long remain unknown. Finding a relatively normal electrocardiogram tracing for a patient several years after a myocardial infarction would not necessarily be predictive of a good long-term prognosis, but finding widespread metastatic carcinoma after opening an abdomen would be immediately conclusive.

Health Care Management Outcomes. For present quality assurance purposes, it is often more practical to assess outcomes categorized by major patient management functions, rather than by the basic outcome classes shown in Table 2.1. The most frequently measured groups include diagnostic, therapeutic, and educational outcomes.

Diagnostic outcomes are the results of the process of data gathering, data analysis, and diagnostic synthesis. The results of such diagnostic processes are conclusions regarding screening, definitive diagnostic labeling, therapeutic planning, or evaluation and prognosis. Assessment of these outcomes usually implies evaluating the validity, necessity, and adequacy of the data acquired and determining the probability of the diagnostic hypothesis subsequently formulated.

Therapeutic outcomes are the results of care processes and include overall patient health status, health problem status, or both. When measured in terms of overall patient health status, such outcomes would comprise increased or decreased longevity; level of general physical, emotional, vocational, or social function; and overall level of comfort, as well as levels of anxiety or concern regarding the health problem itself or the care being provided in managing it. Each of these factors concerns the quality of life of the entire person functioning in a social environment and striving for certain self-defined goals. When measured in terms of health problem status, therapeutic outcomes include specific anatomic status or physiological function improvement, stabilization, or deterioration; status of associated symptoms or signs; or simply the continued presence or absence of the problem. These factors, concerning the status of the health problem itself independent of the status of the entire patient, have been the major outcome concerns of traditional medical care.

Educational outcomes are results of teaching and learning processes that are directly related to health care. They include knowledge or understanding gained, altered attitudes, or changed behavior in either the patient or provider as a result of medical care. The patient may have gathered new facts or insights related to his illness; the provider may have gained information that can be generalized beyond the patient for whom care was provided and may contribute to his understanding of a particular health problem. Patient or provider attitudes might include satisfaction or dissatisfaction resulting from the episode of care; behavioral outcomes might be the patient's acquisition of self-care skills or increased or decreased compliance and the provider's improved skills or greater involvement in community health problems as a result of an episode of care. These factors encompass the results of both diagnostic and therapeutic management processes.

Population Focus. Levels of biological and social organization must likewise be specified in selecting outcomes for assessment so as to indicate the dimension of the problem or the care interaction. Quality of care assessment may focus on the molecular level (elevated serum calcium), cells (malignancy seen in a cervical smear), organ systems (cardiovascular shock), overall health status (the patient's functional ability to return to work), families (emotional disruption of spouse's or children's lives), communities (levels of health), or even on state, regional, or national populations. In an institutional context, however, quality assurance focus on small populations with specified health problems will be most meaningful. By identifying a population group and applying sampling procedures, a limited series of individual assessments can be generalized to the larger population. Also, when the assessment focus is at a higher level of biological or social organization, such as a particular patient population, many intervening variables randomize out and thus need not be measured, allowing for a much broader and more efficient assessment focus.

Failure to recognize correctable family or community determinants of individual impairment is a frequent source of missed opportunities to improve the quality of care. Sexual problems, venereal disease, stress, drug abuse, and learning disorders involve outcomes that reflect social problems as much as individual health problems. Here, proper management, and its assessment, usually require recognition and utilization of community resources. The disease, organ system, and organ level orientation of traditional medical practice tends to ignore care implications at the level of the family or the community.

Also, there are those outcomes of care encompassing health services systems aspects that are aggregates of provider or patient outcomes. They reflect system developments or responses to deficiencies in or requirements of the care process. The lack of primary care in urban or rural areas is an outcome of the lack of regional planning and the failure of medical schools to stress primary or family care; the provision of accessible community care in the form of outpatient clinics is the result of assessment of the availability of physician services to specific populations by which a correctable deficiency of community resources was identified.

On the other hand, while the focus of quality assessment should be the group, assessment measurement must usually be conducted at an individual level. The aggregate of individual outcome data provides the composite outcome for the group. Again, evaluation of overall patient health and functional status often warrants immediate priority. Focused functional measurements at the level of organ systems, organs, or cells are important but often not very meaningful unless used in the context of the patient's total health status. Research findings indicate that there may be little or no correlation between the functioning of the patient as an individual (disability) and the status of his health problem (impairment) in many chronic conditions (Burack, 1965). Many patients with severe organic disease are known to function normally, while others with a mild organic disease are completely incapacitated. If outcomes are assessed at too basic a level of biological organization, the result may be a well-controlled health problem in a completely and unnecessarily incapacitated individual. An unacceptable number of cardiac cripples among children and among those discharged from coronary care units illustrates this point (Bergman and Stamm, 1967; Williamson, 1971).

SUMMARY

This chapter has attempted an overview of various aspects relating to health care outcomes, which should be broadly understood as encompassing any characteristic of patients, health problems, providers, or their interaction in the care process resulting from care provided or required, as measured at one point in time. Application of this outcome definition to quality assurance requires specification of *what* outcome of *what* process at *what* time; explicit assessment of the evidence supporting causal relationships between outcome and health care process, including critical analysis regarding its validity; and consensus on the value of health care outcomes in terms of both their helpful and harmful effects.

In view of the wide range of outcomes that can be identified for study, it is considered essential to select those that are critical for identifying care deficiencies and improvement potential. A procedure for analyzing associated outcome factors was suggested, and several practical considerations were presented for applying this concept to quality assurance.

Finally, practical considerations require that to be useful in most practice settings, quality assurance activity should be based on prior evidence of the efficacy of interventions. Determination of the conclusiveness of the outcome to be measured, focus on overall health care management outcomes that goes beyond the restrictions of the medical record, and recognition of potential popuation benefits or disbenefits for a specific practice setting are additional considerations.

REFERENCES

Bergman, A.B., and Stamm, S.J. 1967. Morbidity of cardiac nondisease in school children. *N Engl J Med* 276:1008-13.

Burack, B. 1965. Interdisciplinary classification for the aged. *J Chronic Dis* 18:1059-64.

Delbecq, A.L.; Van de Ven, A.; and Gustafson, D.H. 1975. *Group Techniques for Program Planning. Guide to Normal Group and Delphi Processes.* Glenview, Ill.: Scott, Foresman.

Emlet, H.E., Jr.; Williamson, J.W.; Casey, I.; and Davis, J.L. 1971. *Estimating Health Care Benefits and Required Resources.* Vol. 1, *Summary.* Falls Church, Va.: Analytic Services.

Goldner, M.G.; Knatterud, G.L.; and Prout, T.E. 1971. Effects of hypoglycemic agents on vascular complications in patients with adult-onset diabetes. Pt. 3: Clinical implications of UGDP results. *JAMA* 218:1400-10.

Knatterud, G.L.; Meinert, C.L.; Klimt, C.R.; Osborne, R.K.; and Martin, D.B. 1971. Effects of hypoglycemic agents on vascular complications in patients with adult-onset diabetes. Pt. 4: A preliminary report on Phenformin results. *JAMA* 217:777-84.

Kohn, R., and White, K.L., eds. 1976. *Health Care—An International Study.* London: Oxford University Press.

National Research Council. 1969. *Drug Efficacy Study.* Final Report to the Commission of Food and Drugs from the Division of Medical Sciences. Washington: National Academy of Sciences.

Neuhauser, D., and Johnson, E. 1974. Managerial response to new health care technology: Coronary artery bypass surgery. In *The Management of Health Care*, Abernathy, W.J., Sheldon, A., and Prahalad, C.K., eds., pp. 205-13. Cambridge, Mass: Ballinger.

Payne, B.C.; Lyons, T.F.; Dwarshins, L.; Kolton, M.; and Morris, W. 1976. *Quality of Medical Care: Evaluation and Improvement.* Health Services Monograph Series T40. Chicago: Hospital Research and Education Trust.

Starfield, B. 1974. Measurement of outcome: A proposed scheme. *Milbank Mem Fund Q* 52:39-50.

University Group Diabetes Program. 1970. A study of the effects of hypoglycemic agents on vascular complications in patients with adult-onset diabetes. Pt. 1: Design, methods and baseline results; pt. 2: Mortality results. *Diabetes* 19(suppl. 2): 747-85; 787-830.

Veterans Administration Cooperative Study Group on Antihypertensive Agents. 1967. Effects of treatment on morbidity in hypertension. Results in patients with diastolic blood pressure averaging 115 through 129 mm Hg. *JAMA* 202:1028-34.

———. 1970. Effects of treatment on morbidity in hypertension. Pt. 2: Results in patients with diastolic blood pressure averaging 90 through 114 mm Hg. *JAMA* 213:1143-52.

———. 1972. Effects of treatment on morbidity in hypertension. Pt. 3: Influence of age, diastolic pressure and prior cardiovascular disease; further analysis of side effects. *Circulation* 45:991-1004.

Williamson, J.W. 1971. Evaluating the quality of patient care—a strategy relating outcome and process assessment. *JAMA* 218:564-69.

Williamson, J.W.; Braswell, H.R.; Horn, S.D.; and Lohmeyer, S. 1978. Priority setting in quality assurance: Reliability of staff judgment in medical institutions. *Med Care* (in press).

Chapter 3

The Estimation of Achievable Health Care Benefit

The practice of medicine requires a continual series of priority decisions. A large and varied range of patients, health problems, and available resources must be coordinated within extremely narrow constraints of time and effort. Each patient provides a challenge as to how much data to collect, what diagnostic possibilities to consider, what therapeutic modalities to utilize, when to seek greater expertise by consultation or referral, and what proportion of effort to apply to caring as opposed to curing functions. Similar priorities must be developed to plan the use of time for practice assessment or continuing medical education and to allocate resources within the framework of health planning at state, regional, or national levels. A realistic determination of health or health economic benefits achievable but not presently being achieved, whether in health care generally or in medical practice specifically, can make an important contribution to the setting of priorities for resource allocation and for program evaluation and development.

Such decisions can be made more meaningful if they are based on a clear statement of that which is realistic and attainable, in conditions obtaining for a specific provider and in relation to a given patient or health problem. In the following, the main emphasis in developing the concept of achievable health care benefit and its correlate, the achievable benefit that is not achieved, will be in regard to the setting of priorities for quality assurance in personal health services. It is argued, and can be supported by evidence from a number of quality assurance projects using this approach, that the concept of achievable benefits not achieved (ABNA) encourages quality assurance planners to make explicit their assumptions regarding how much of what type of care benefit is possible within the constraints of both present knowledge and available resources (Williamson et al., 1975; Williamson, 1971). Equally important, it encourages them to make explicit those assumptions of provider and patient values that are implicit in defining benefit and in determining how much of what type of care warrants immediate effort.

Further, the concept can be applied to any outcome aspect, whether diagnostic, therapeutic, educational, or economic, and defined in relation to any group in the care interaction process, whether patient, potential patient, provider, or society as a whole. It directs quality assurance to those areas where benefit is considered achievable and, by definition, excludes areas where evidence of the efficacy of interventions, or the potential for improved effectiveness or efficiency of health services, is lacking. At all levels of practice, this means that only those content areas that are considered capable of significant improvement at the present time and under realistic resource constraints are eligible for quality assurance study.

The determination of achievable benefit not achieved has become practicable due to the development of small group estimation techniques (see also Chapter 5), which permit quality assurance staff to define and even quantify improvement potential in a relatively short time. The process of formulating this measure of benefit not achieved often proves valuable from an educational point of view. Providers gain an understanding of basic conceptual tools that can be applied, not only to quality assurance projects, but to their practice and to their other educational interests as well. In the author's experience, these formal procedures call attention to such critical issues as the validity of scientific knowledge, the limits of human perception (as reflected in the extent of clinical observer error even among experts), and the scarcity of documented research evidence on the efficacy of interventions.

HEALTH CARE BENEFIT

The significance of the concept of health care benefit, and of the derived concepts of achievable benefit and achievable benefit not achieved, lies in the fact that they are fundamental to most decisions on priorities in clinical practice, quality assurance, and health policy development. Health care benefit in this context refers to those outcomes of health care that, by the criteria discussed in Chapter 2, have an overall positive value and for which there is reasonable evidence of a causal relationship with antecedent care processes.

A useful application of the concept of achievable benefits of health care relates to three basic quality assurance indicators—the efficacy, effectiveness, and efficiency of health care. Here, efficacy is the maximum benefit that can be achieved by a given intervention, effectiveness denotes the net benefit of care achieved under actual conditions of practice as measured against the potential for accomplishment, and efficiency is the relation to benefits achieved of the costs of care expended in terms of money, human and physical resources, and time. By extension, the concept of achievable benefit not achieved indicates that benefit of health care that is possible, given the state of medical science and local conditions of care, but that is not being attained, whether due to insufficient provider performance or to misallocation or inefficient use of available resources.

For the majority of purposes of quality assurance, the recipients of health care are populations or subgroups of populations. In order to quantify the health care benefits potentially available to them, it is necessary to determine both the average benefit per person and the number of persons involved. A similar level of benefit might be achievable for problems involving considerable disability per person but relatively few people, on the one hand, as for problems involving comparatively little disability per person but large numbers of people, on the other. For example, in malignant melanoma, early diagnosis and treatment can be life saving. The potential benefit from health care for the small number of people affected by this relatively rare disease is large and perhaps comparable to that for a more common problem such as osteoarthritis, for which improvement potential is much smaller, but which affects a far larger subgroup of the population. Thus, in setting assessment priorities, the number of patients who might benefit within a given practice setting must be considered, in addition to the potential benefit for each patient.

Also, locally available health care resources often do not allow attainment of the full extent of benefits as demonstrated under research conditions. Allocation of resources demands that relative priorities be established reflecting local patient and provider values. If cardiovascular problems receive high priority, highly trained cardiologists may be attracted, much sophisticated equipment purchased, and perhaps expensive surgical capability developed. The capability of managing cardiovascular problems in a community might thus closely approximate maximum achievable benefits, at the cost of limiting the capability for managing other problems, e.g., by reducing the priority of mental health care, rehabilitation, health education, and preventive medicine programs. Such offsetting dis-benefits must be recognized not only for resource allocation but also in planning quality assurance activities, especially in the setting of assessment standards.

Theoretically at least, this consideration makes the establishment of universally applicable health care standards an extremely difficult if not unattainable goal. Thus, local groups should formulate, within the limits of demonstrated efficacy, standards that reflect the extent of benefit that can reasonably be attained with available health care resources in their facility or community. This extent of reasonable benefit will then provide the denominator for defining the effectiveness of health care. The attainable benefit will vary from facility to facility, and possibly from community to community, depending upon available resources, professional capacity, and local values. Setting the limits of achievable benefits, therefore, requires that the value systems of both providers and consumers of health care be made explicit. While providers express their values in terms of qualifications and interests of personnel selected and facilities acquired, consumers express their individual values by selecting a given facility when requesting care and by the degree of compliance in following the care recommendations received; likewise, community values are expressed in authorizing public funds for specific programs. Reasonable estimates of achievable benefits must incorporate all such value aspects. Whether and how this is done may be an important determinant of ultimate success in quality assurance.

THE CONCEPT OF ACHIEVABLE BENEFIT NOT ACHIEVED AS A TOOL OF QUALITY ASSURANCE

Achievable Diagnostic Benefit Not Achieved

Valid diagnostic outcomes are essential for positive patient health outcomes, to the extent that accurate and complete formulation of the health problem is a prerequisite of effective therapeutic management where efficacious therapy is available. The extent of health improvement achievable by competent diagnostic management is a direct function of the validity, necessity, and adequacy of diagnostic information; validity being the accuracy with which diagnostic information reflects the patient's health problem and the characteristics influencing it, and necessity and adequacy referring to the extent to which required diagnostic information is obtained and nonessential information is excluded.

The most practical quantification of achievable diagnostic benefit is thus in terms of the validity, necessity, and adequacy of diagnostic information as collected, analyzed, and synthesized by experts. For quality assurance purposes, achievable diagnostic benefit not achieved can be determined by comparing diagnostic information formulated by any given provider with that compiled by experts or available from a criterion variable. As illustrated in Figure 3.1, the results of the application by a specific provider group of a specific diagnostic mode to a specific patient population can be expressed in terms of patients who have true positive, false positive, true negative, and false negative diagnoses. Diagnostic benefit is then defined as the extent to which true positive and true negative diagnoses have been made and false positive and false negative diagnoses avoided. In this scheme, achievable benefits not achieved can be expressed as the percentage of false negative and of false positive diagnostic results, computed as follows:

$$\text{Percent False Negatives} = \frac{\text{False Negatives}}{\text{False Negatives} + \text{True Positives}} (100)$$

$$\text{Percent False Positives} = \frac{\text{False Positives}}{\text{False Positives} + \text{True Positives}} (100)$$

Note that this computation of the percentage of false negatives and of false positives avoids the confounding effect of health problem prevalence as reflected in the number of true negatives. By not using the latter in either denominator, a more stable and meaningful rate is obtained.

The determination of deficient diagnostic benefit is illustrated in Figure 3.2 (Galen and Gambino, 1975), showing the results obtained by research cardiologists who examined 1,000 patients, verifying the presence of left ventricular hypertrophy in 50, and by an independent group of community hospital cardiologists, who examined only electrocardiograms for the same 1,000 patients. Based on electrocardiogram evidence alone, the community cardiologists missed 21 of 50 hypertrophic patients, yielding a false negative rate of 42 percent (21/50 $\times$ 100) and diagnosed 57 as having left ventricular hypertrophy, of whom 28 did not in fact have this condition, yielding a false positive rate of 49 percent (28/57 $\times$ 100). Thus, if the

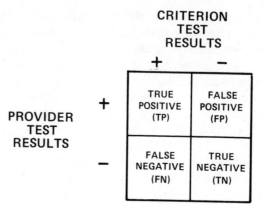

Figure 3.1. Theoretical model for determination of achievable diagnostic benefit not achieved by comparing criterion test with provider test results.

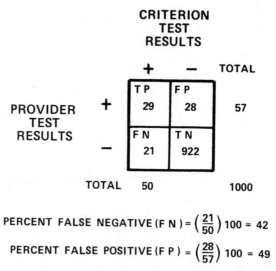

$$\text{PERCENT FALSE NEGATIVE (F N)} = \left(\frac{21}{50}\right) 100 = 42$$

$$\text{PERCENT FALSE POSITIVE (F P)} = \left(\frac{28}{57}\right) 100 = 49$$

Figure 3.2. Application of theoretical model to the determination of deficient diagnostic benefit in provider diagnoses of left ventricular hypertrophy (Source: Galen and Gambino, 1975).

results obtained by the research cardiologists can be considered to represent achievable diagnostic benefit, then less than half of this benefit was actually achieved on the basis of electrocardiogram data alone; it is not unreasonable to assume that analogous results will often be reached in the day-to-day practice of medicine. Accepting that there is efficacious treatment for the hypertension and/or heart failure probably encompassed by these 50 patients, the diagnostic deficiency in terms of false negatives could indicate considerable preventable health impairment that is not being prevented or, in terms of false positives, considerable health disbenefit for those receiving potent but unnecessary drugs.

Much of clinical practice encompasses considerable diagnostic benefit not achieved, a subject reviewed by Garland (1949), Kilpatrick (1963), and Galen and Gambino (1975). The number of errors occurring under skilled, experienced professionals has been found to be shocking in many instances. Patient history data are frequently of poor quality, sometimes due to directive questioning instead of open-ended methods or to questions that are not intelligible to the patient or elicit ambiguous replies. Cochrane's studies of history taking from coal miners in England, in which such items as "pain," "dyspnea," or "cough" were elicited, showed that the extent of observer interpretation applied and the accuracy of the information obtained varied considerably among different observers (Cochrane, Chapman, and Oldham, 1951).

Physical examination data are notoriously unreliable in studies of such problems as determination of nutritional status of children (Derryberry, 1938) and emphysema in adults (Fletcher, 1952). A well-known study in which 1,000 eleven year old children were examined for diseased tonsils revealed that 611 had already had a tonsillectomy; when the remaining 389 were examined, 174 were recommended for tonsillectomy, and the remaining 215 were found to be healthy. When this "healthy" group was examined by a second group of physicians, 99 were recommended for tonsillectomy and 116 found healthy. When this "healthy" group was in turn examined by a third group of physicians, 51 were recommended for tonsillectomy and 65 found healthy (American Child Health Association, 1934). Kilpatrick (1963) comments that it was fortunate for the remaining patients that the supply of physician panels ran out at this point.

Laboratory data studies have revealed similar problems. Davies (1958) reported that a team of ten physicians, nine of whom were especially qualified in cardiology, were asked each to read the same 100 electrocardiograms, including 50 showing evidence of myocardial infarction, 25 with other abnormalities, and 25 normals. Comparison of the results among the nine cardiologists revealed serious discrepancies in the interpretation of 20 percent of the tracings; further, the physicians disagreed with themselves on one in eight readings of the same tracings two weeks later. It has been repeatedly reported that any one chest specialist may miss as many as 20 to 25 percent of chest films showing abnormalities, the missed lesions being randomly distributed and not related to the size or description of the lesion (Kilpatrick, 1963; Cochrane and Garland, 1952).

A 1975 study showed that 800 technicians in 300 laboratories missed 30 percent of test slides of cervical smears strongly indicating adenocarcinoma of the cervix, while the pathologists in the same laboratories missed close to 37 percent on the same slides (LaMotte, 1975). LaMotte has obtained even more disconcerting data from the Laboratory Licensing and Proficiency Testing Division of the Center for Disease Control, which conducted a study to determine differences in the validity of test results identifying drug abuse substances (narcotics, barbiturates, or amphetamines), depending upon whether or not the laboratory staff knew that their performance was being evaluated. Among a random sample of 24 laboratories participating in the testing program, the average score for the 21 laboratories from whom complete data were obtained indicated 96 percent accuracy, with a range of 71 to 100 percent, when the specimen was known to be part of a proficiency test sample sent by the center. On the other hand, when the other half of the same set of specimens were sent to local physicians who submitted them to the same laboratories as though they were from their own practice, the average score dropped to 50 percent, with a range of 0 to 100 percent. This is a dramatic illustration of achievable diagnostic benefit not achieved.

Achievable Therapeutic Benefit
Not Achieved

Achievable therapeutic benefit in relation to patient health can be defined and quantified in terms of the demonstrated effect of therapy on the course of a given impairment over time. Figure 3.3 is an illustration of this as applied to myocardial infarction. The projected course with and without care is plotted. Therapeutic benefit as shown in this figure represents the extent of achievable reduction in impairment by a given therapy. Comparing the course of the patient's functional impairment in the absence of professional care (solid line) with its probable course under reasonable professional care (broken line), it is evident that the smaller the distance between the two curves, the smaller the benefit achievable from therapy; the greater the distance, the greater the benefit. Conversely, achievable benefit not achieved in relation to therapeutic management is established by comparing the course of patient health impairment resulting from care actually provided (dotted line in Figure 3.3) to the course established for conditions of reasonable care. A crude measure of

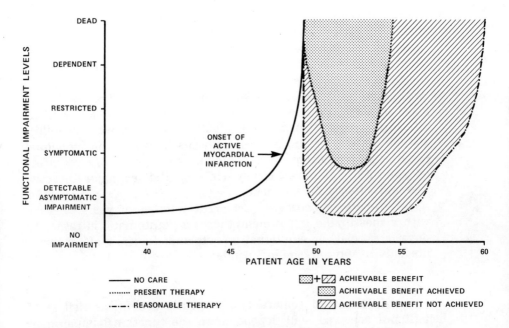

Figure 3.3. Determination of deficient therapeutic benefit in terms of life years lost and of decreased function years, by comparing three modalities of care (no care, present therapy, reasonable therapy).

achievable therapeutic benefit can then be provided by a tabulation of additional years at any level of lesser impairment. In the example in Figure 3.3, an achievable benefit of approximately 12 additional years of life was possible, but only 5 years were actually achieved; further, approximately 8 symptom-free years might have been achieved, but only 2 were realized by the care provided. The health benefit not achieved—i.e., that was lost due to decreased longevity or to years spent impaired or disabled—can thus be defined by the number of life years falling into one of the following categories (Williamson, Alexander, and Miller, 1968; Berdit and Williamson, 1973, as augmented by Gross, 1977):

- *Life years lost*—The number of years between birth and age 100 that were lost by death.
- *Dependent years*—The number of years in dependent status, defined as requiring mechanical or human assistance for activities of daily living (such as eating, dressing, toilet function) and being unable to perform one's major life activity (school, work).

- *Restricted years*—The number of years in which the individual was unable to perform his major life activity (whether play, school, work, or active retirement) but was able to manage activities of daily living (toilet function, ambulation, eating) with minimal assistance.
- *Social, emotional and/or physical symptom years*—The number of years of social isolation, conflict, or other social impairment significantly greater than the individual's previous proven capability and desire, and/or the number of years in which the individual experiences physical or emotional signs or symptoms of discomfort or reduced functional efficiency while maintaining major life activities and self-care independence.
- *Asymptomatic impairment years*—The number of years of living with a measurable impairment that is asymptomatic in regard to physical, social, or emotional aspects and does not affect major life activity and self-care independence.

The quantification of achievable therapeutic benefit, as well as of benefit not achieved, will depend upon the functional impairment scale applied. Here, ordinal or cardinal scales may be used. The ordinal scale is a rank order scale in which each successive level indicates more impairment than the preceding level, without specifying how much impairment is involved. The cardinal (or interval) scale is a rank order scale in which each level not only indicates more impairment but specifies how much more. Because of the problems inherent in reducing all impairments to common units of measurements, universally applicable cardinal scales are very difficult to develop. Among the more interesting research in this area is that of Rosser and Watts in England, using fiscal data from court awards based on the disability of the plaintiff to establish scale intervals (Rosser and Watts, 1972). They have developed a functional ratio scale with an absolute zero and a known interval (ratio scale). The studies of Torrance, Thomas, and Sackett (1972) and of Fanshel and Bush (1970) provide other examples of health interval scale development in the United States and Canada.

Several recent reviews (Gross, 1977; Coles et al., 1976; Chen and Bryant, 1975; Goldsmith, 1973), as well as abstracts from the clearinghouse on health indexes of the Health Resources Administration, provide detailed analyses of the state of the art of health scale development. One of the more promising instruments is the Sickness Impact Profile (Gilson et al., 1975). Overall, however, few methods have proven reliable, valid, and practical for current quality assurance uses.

DETERMINING THE POTENTIAL FOR IMPROVEMENT

Bearing in mind the definitions discussed previously (see also Chapter 1), the three basic assessment indicators of quality of care—efficacy, effectiveness, and efficiency—can provide useful quality assurance standards for the identification and specification of achievable benefits.

Efficacy Index

It has been stated repeatedly in this discussion that in order to be useful, assessment of quality of care must not include formal study of the efficacy of care interventions, but rather that acceptable proof of efficacy is a prerequisite of subsequent quality assurance effort. However, an efficacy index can be formulated to provide the basis for determining the achievable benefit of care (Figure 3.4). This efficacy index refers to that portion of the maximum conceivable benefit of care that is actually achievable. As related to health, the maximum conceivable benefit would indicate the desirable, but usually unattainable, elimination of all patient or population disability, impairment, or risk that is expected in the absence of medical interventions. The achievable benefit of care would then be reflected in assessment standards which take into consideration both the state of the art and local provider and consumer values as expressed in terms of available facilities; levels of expertise, particularly in regard to secondary and tertiary levels of care; and reasonable expectations regarding patient compliance compatible with current lifestyles. This efficacy index is computed as the rate of

$$\frac{\text{Achievable Benefit}}{\text{Maximum Conceivable Benefit}} (100)$$

A practical example of the usefulness of such an index for quality assurance at the community level would be in regard to the detection and treatment of Group A beta hemolytic streptococcal infections, where health benefit can be defined in terms of primary prevention of first attacks of rheumatic fever in a metropolitan area. Extrapolating from epidemiological data reported by Gordis and Markowitz

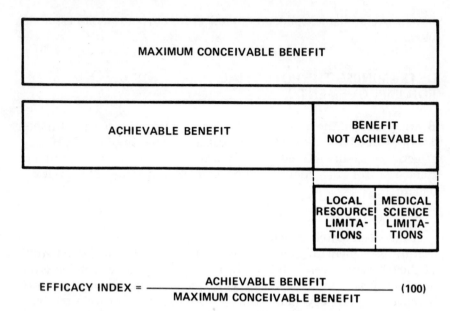

$$\text{EFFICACY INDEX} = \frac{\text{ACHIEVABLE BENEFIT}}{\text{MAXIMUM CONCEIVABLE BENEFIT}} \quad (100)$$

Figure 3.4. An index of the efficacy of health care, expressed as the rate of achievable benefit of care to the maximum conceivable benefit, where the portion of benefit not achievable is determined by local resource limitations and the state of the art of medicine.

(1972), it can be theorized that given the present state of the art of medical science, most of a five year total of 261 cases of first attacks of rheumatic fever in a metropolitan area could be prevented under ideal conditions of care given unlimited resources—namely, an intensive community health education program to achieve complete reporting of all throat infections in children and adolescents, plus taking throat cultures for all cases of pharyngitis thus reported; followup cultures of asymptomatic siblings of patients with positive cultures revealing beta hemolytic streptococcus; adequate physician management and patient compliance resulting in a full ten day course of treatment with penicillin (or erythromycin if allergic to penicillin) for those having a positive culture; and followup cultures to determine eradication of the pathogens.

However, community values of both providers and consumers of health care as expressed in available resources, facilities, and patient compliance levels would probably not favor the effort and financial expenditures required to obtain theoretically possible levels of total primary prevention. Consequently, an adjustment must be made to reflect a more realistic goal for health outcomes. Thus, if only those symptomatic pharyngitis patients contacting a physician were to receive throat cultures, if a limited health education effort were made to teach parents that rheumatic fever can be prevented by detecting and eradicating streptococcus throat infections, if asymptomatic siblings of those having a positive culture were cultured as well, and if adequate antibiotic treatment were provided to all patients having a positive culture, perhaps approximately 100 cases (38 percent of 261) could be prevented with reasonable effort. This extrapolation is based on data from the Gordis and Markowitz study (1972), on the following assumptions:

- Obtaining cultures for siblings of patients having positive throat cultures would yield 13 cases (15 percent) from among the 89 in the group of 261 first attacks of rheumatic fever who had been asymptomatic prior to onset (negative history for clinical respiratory infection);
- Providing a limited community program of health education for the 83 among the 261 first rheumatic fever attacks who had been symptomatic in terms of an upper respiratory infection but had not seen a physician for care would yield another 21 cases (25 percent); and
- All 88 of the group who had been symptomatic and had contacted a physician were cultured and group A beta hemolytic streptococcus was detected.

This would yield a total of 122 cases with positive cultures. Finally, assuming that with reasonable effort it were possible to achieve at least 80 percent eradication of Group A beta hemolytic streptococcus—by use of intramuscular bicillin and assuming minimal treatment failures—98 of the 261 first attacks of rheumatic fever identified by Gordis and Markowitz might be prevented. For purposes of computing an efficacy index, therefore, if the benefit to be achieved in terms of primary prevention is assumed to be 261 cases, then achievable benefit adjusted for local conditions might reasonably encompass at least the 98 cases extrapolated above—an efficacy index of 38 percent.

In other words, a practicable goal for community quality assurance activity might be a 38 percent reduction in the incidence of rheumatic fever expected in the absence of preventive care. Also implied is that an additional improvement of up to 62 percent of cases of primary prevention of rheumatic fever would be theoretically possible if the community, both consumers and providers, elected to make the necessary effort. Obviously, such an effort would be costly, involve considerable time and a coordinated effort not only to educate patients but to educate providers as well, and finally, require communitywide health care systems changes such as providing throat cultures without a physician visit. The main utility of such an efficacy index would lie in indicating the extent of possible health care benefit for specific patient populations, health problems, or interventions, given optimum conditions of management, and in identifying areas where increased benefit would be achievable by greater resource expenditure and more concerted effort than could be reasonably expected from present health resources and management.

Effectiveness Index
The net accomplishment of health care provided under conditions of local practice can then similarly be quantified by formulating an index of effectiveness, computed as the rate of

$$\frac{\text{Benefit achieved}}{\text{Achievable benefit}} (100)$$

where the scope of the benefit will depend on the target benefit desired in terms of either individuals or populations.

Here, benefits actually achieved constitute the numerator, and achievable benefits the denominator for computing effectiveness; the extent of achievable benefit not achieved then provides the major target for improvement action (Figure 3.5). The illustrative computation based on extrapolation from epidemiological data by Gordis and Markowitz (1972) indicated that for first attacks of rheumatic heart disease in a metropolitan city, an efficacy index of 38 percent might be reasonable. In other words, the expected incidence of this disease could be reduced by one-third given an improved primary prevention effort involving both providers and consumers of health care. Applying these figures to the incidence of first attacks of rheumatic fever in the 5 to 19 year old age group (28.5 per 100,000) reported by the National Health Survey, Baltimore Region, for 1935-1936 (Collins, 1947), achievable health benefit of modern preventive care might be a reduction in this incidence by 10.8 per 100,000 in this age group (38 percent × 28.5).

This figure would then provide the denominator for an effectiveness index to be applied in assessing health care benefits in fact achieved. Gordis and Markowitz have measured a subsequent first

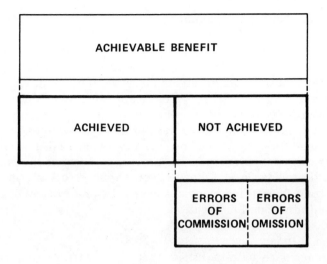

$$\text{EFFECTIVENESS INDEX} = \frac{\text{BENEFIT ACHIEVED}}{\text{ACHIEVABLE BENEFIT}} (100)$$

Figure 3.5. An index of the effectiveness of health care, expressed as the rate of achievable benefit not achieved to achievable benefit, where the portion of benefit not achieved is attributable to harmful effects of care provided or to helpful care omitted.

attack incidence for rheumatic fever in Baltimore for the period 1960–1964. By then, the incidence had dropped to 21.0 per 100,000, that is, a gain of 7.5 per 100,000 had been realized, probably due mainly to the availability of penicillin. Assuming adequate evidence supporting the attribution of the improvement to modern health care, the following effectiveness index could be computed for this hypothetical quality assurance topic:

$$\frac{\text{Benefit Achieved}}{\text{Achievable Benefit}} = \frac{7.5/100,000}{10.8/100,000}(100) = 69.4 \text{ percent}$$

implying that, although significant improvement was achieved, much more remains to be done within the bounds of what is judged reasonable performance. Quality assurance effort should be directed at establishing the reasons for the deficiency and at determining what steps might be most effectively taken to improve outcomes.

Further, achievable benefit not achieved can be attributed to errors of omission and of commission, where the latter are those unnecessary and harmful interventions that detract from achievable benefit and the former lie in the failure to provide an efficacious intervention when it is indicated. In determining achievable benefit not achieved, both types of errors must be considered. Correctable problems might include errors of omission, such as failure to obtain throat cultures for patients at risk of streptococcal infection, to follow up on abnormal laboratory results, or to provide patients with specific instructions on medication. Any or all of these might be indicators of ineffectiveness in the provision of care at the individual patient and provider level. Likewise, correctable errors of commission might detract from effectiveness, such as the prescription of ineffective or contraindicated medication.

Efficiency Index

What remains to be established, then, is the efficiency with which the net accomplishment of health care (here, a reduction in the rate of first attacks of rheumatic fever in the 5 to 19 year old population of a metropolitan area) has been achieved in relation to costs in terms of money, human and physical resources, and time. This efficiency index is computed as the rate of

$$\frac{\text{Cost related to benefit achieved}}{\text{Total costs of care}} (100)$$

which is obtained by dividing total health care costs spent to obtain a given benefit into that portion related to health benefits achieved (necessary costs) and the portion that was not so related (unnecessary costs). The unnecessary cost component can be further divided into costs of harmful care and costs of inutile care (Figure 3.6). For example, if a physician prescribes a combination of penicillin, tetracycline, and antihistamines for a patient with streptococcal pharyngitis, the cost of the tetracycline would be for a contraindicated, potentially damaging agent; the cost of the antihistamine for an inutile but probably harmless agent; and the cost of the penicillin for a helpful agent. Thus, if the penicillin cost is $10.00, the tetracycline $12.00, and the antihistamine $3.00, the efficiency index would be computed as

$$\frac{\text{Cost related to benefit achieved}}{\text{Total cost of care}} = \frac{10}{25} (100) = 40 \text{ percent}$$

in relation to drug treatment of this particular health problem.

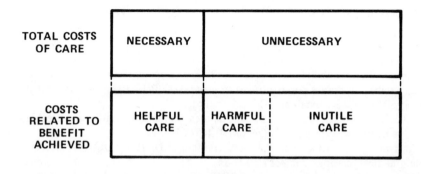

$$\text{EFFICIENCY INDEX} = \frac{\text{COSTS RELATED TO BENEFIT ACHIEVED}}{\text{TOTAL COSTS OF CARE}} \quad (100)$$

Figure 3.6. An index of the efficiency of health care, expressed as the rate of the cost of care related to benefit achieved to the total costs of care, where the portion of cost unrelated to benefit was expended on harmful and inutile care.

The significance of efficacy, effectiveness, and efficiency indicators of quality of care for assessment and improvement planning can thus be summarized by formulating a relationship where efficacy, adjusted for the state of the art and local facilities, sets the boundaries of health care benefit to be achieved and provides the denominator (or assessment standard) for determining effectiveness of health care and where benefits actually achieved, expressed in terms of cost, provide the numerator for determining its efficiency.

SUMMARY

This chapter has delineated the concept of health care benefit, with emphasis on quality assurance applications. The related concepts of achievable benefit of care and achievable benefit not achieved have been discussed in relation both to diagnostic and therapeutic outcomes of health care and to the classic assessment indicators of quality of care—efficacy, effectiveness, and efficiency. The latter have been used to construct indexes for measuring performance and improvement potential, taking into account the state of the art of medicine and actual conditions of clinical practice. The assessment of health care outcomes in terms of these three functional indexes has practical implications not only for quality assurance in personal health care, but also for health policy formulation, as the principles illustrated should apply with equal validity at individual, community, or national levels.

REFERENCES

American Child Health Association. 1934. *Physical Defects; The Pathway to Correction.* New York: American Child Health Association.

Berdit, M., and Williamson, J.W. 1973. Function limitation scale for measuring health outcomes. In *Health Status Indexes*, R.L. Berg, ed., pp. 59–65. Chicago: Hospital Research and Education Trust.

Chen, M.K., and Bryant, B.E. 1975. The measurement of health—a critical and selective overview. *Internat J Epidemiol* 4:257–64.

Cochrane, A.L.; Chapman, P.J.; and Oldham, P.D. 1951. Observer's error in taking medical histories. *Lancet* i:1007–09.

Cochrane, A.L., and Garland, L.H. 1952. Observer errors in the interpretation of chest films. Lancet ii:505–09.

Coles, J.M.; Davison A.J.; Neal, D.M.; and Wickings, H.I. 1976. A comparison of three health status indicators. *Internat J Epidemiol* 5:237–46.

Collins, S.D. 1947. The incidence of rheumatic fever as recorded in general morbidity surveys of families. *Public Health Rep*, Suppl. 198.

Davies, L.G. 1958. Observer variation in reports on electrocardiograms. *Br Heart J* 20:153–61.

Derryberry, M. 1938. Reliability of medical judgment on malnutrition. *Public Health Rep* 53:263–68.

Fanshel, S., and Bush, J.W. 1970. A health-status index and its application to health-services outcomes. *Operations Research* 18:1021–66.

Fletcher, C.M. 1952. The clinical diagnosis of pulmonary emphysema: an experimental study. *Proc R Soc Med* 45:577–84.

Galen, R.S., and Gambino, S.R. 1975. *Beyond Normality: The Predictive Value and Efficiency of Medical Diagnosis.* New York: Wiley.

Garland, L.H. 1949. On the scientific evaluation of diagnostic procedures. *Radiology* 52:309–27.

Gilson, B.S.; Gilson, J.S.; Bergner, M.; Bobbitt, R.A.; Kressel, S.; Pollard, W.E.; and Vesselago, M. 1975. The sickness impact profile—development of an outcome measure of health care. *Am J Public Health* 65:1304–10.

Goldsmith, S. 1973. A reevaluation of health status indicators. *Health Serv Rep* 88:937–41.

Gordis, L., and Markowitz, M. 1972. Environmental determinants in rheumatic fever prevention. In *Streptococci and Streptococcal Diseases—Recognition, Understanding, and Management*, L.W. Wannamaker and J.M. Matsen, eds., pp. 595–609. New York and London: Academic Press.

Gross, R. 1977. Outcome measures of medical care: development and evaluation of a functional status measure for quality assurance. Master of Science thesis, Johns Hopkins University School of Hygiene and Public Health.

Kilpatrick, G.S. 1963. Observer error in medicine. *J Med Educ* 38:38–43.

Lamotte, L. 1975. Personal communication.

Rosser, R.M., and Watts, V.C. 1972. The measurement of hospital output. *Internat J Epidemiol* 1:361–68.

Torrance, G.W.; Thomas, W.H.; and Sackett, D.L. 1972. A utility maximization model for evaluation of health care programs. *Health Serv Res* 7:118–33.

Williamson, J.W. 1971. Evaluating the quality of patient care—a strategy relating outcome and process assessment. *JAMA* 218:564-69.

Williamson, J.W.; Alexander, J.; and Miller, G.E. 1968. Priorities in patient care research and continuing medical education. *JAMA* 204:93-98.

Williamson, J.W.; Aronovitch, S.; Simonson, L.; Ramirez, C.; and Kelly, D. 1975. Health accounting: an outcome based system of quality assurance: illustrative application to hypertension. *Bull NY Acad Med* 51:727-38.

Chapter 4

Expanding the Boundaries of Medical Practice and Health Care: Points of Emphasis for Quality Assurance

To apply assessment and improvement concepts with a view to increasing the effectiveness and efficiency of current performance, specific health care content must be identified. This task is especially important because the potential for significant health improvement or for a reduction in care expenditures may well be curtailed by traditional views of medical care and the limits of its responsibilities. Emphasis on advanced organic disease or on crisis events where drugs and surgery are the major interventions required often leads to neglect of preventive care, patient health education, or psychosocial counseling. If substantial improvement of health or other outcomes of care is the ultimate goal, the selection of specific aspects to be assessed is likely to be more important than how the assessment is accomplished; in the long run, assessment content will prove of greater significance than assessment procedures.

The following is an overview of the basic elements involved in any health care transaction—the patient, the health problem, and the provider of care. It attempts to indicate a range of assessment topics that may have immediate potential for achieving improvement and to go beyond the traditional focus on organic medical disease, which tends to neglect specific local characteristics of patients and providers or their interaction in the care process.

THE PATIENT

Understanding the consumers of medical care apart from their health problems is essential in designing outcome assessment studies. Each patient presents many characteristics that affect the manifestation of his problem, the manner in which he deals with it, and the type and significance of related outcomes. Many variables—age, physical condition, education, occupation, geographic or genetic factors—may affect whether a person is likely to acquire a given health problem or how early in its course he may be aware of its presence. Attitudes may affect whether and how soon medical care is sought. There are many reasons why a patient may or may not provide the physician with sufficient and accurate diagnostic information. Financial status or understanding of the patient's role in health care may determine whether the prescribed treatment will be followed, and each of these variables may have an effect on the eventual health outcome. Also, certain patient characteristics may change as a result of care; these may well provide profitable topics for outcome assessment, such as the understanding of health problems or attitudes toward physicians, and indicate correctable determinants of deficient health results.

Patient characteristics and factors, considered apart from health problems as such, have been categorized in various ways; a useful approach by Lerner (1977) divides these factors into internal or endogenous and external or exogenous factors, although it is recognized that in practice these factors may overlap considerably.

Endogenous Patient Factors

Five major factors may be considered endogenous to the individual: biological, genetic, affective, cognitive, and behavioral attributes. Among biological factors, age and sex are major determinants of health services use and of health outcomes. Vital statistics abstracts and other sources show that impairment and health services use increase directly with age and that causes of morbidity and mortality are significantly different among the age groups (Wilder, 1972; Ranofsky, 1973); also, many health problems are more prevalent in one sex than the other. Hypertension, for example, is more common among males, and the most common hospital discharge diagnosis for males in 1968 was disorders of the digestive system; for females, not surprisingly, the most common diagnosis was deliveries and complications of pregnancy and childbirth (Ranofsky, 1973). Assessment studies focusing on health status differentials by sex or by age, e.g., for those over 65 who frequently seek health care, might indicate significant achievable benefit in terms of matching resources to specific population needs or of measuring physician skills in distinguishing normal from abnormal patterns.

Psychomotor factors such as visual, auditory, and tactile abilities and muscular strength and coordination may determine a patient's gross level of function. This and the degree of dependence on others for activities of daily living may be major factors in the patient's ability to communicate and to cooperate in his own medical care. Particularly in rehabilitative care, these are important evaluation factors. While genetic factors cannot for the most part be altered by medical care, for quality assessment purposes the desirability and effectiveness of eugenic management might be studied. The result of genetic counseling to prevent the conception of children who might have serious hereditary defects is an outcome of care that can be measured by establishing the birth rates for children from high risk genetic unions (Fraser, 1973).

Affective, cognitive, and behavioral factors are likewise important characteristics endogenous to the patient and related to health. They may affect diagnoses of mental illness as well as general patient management. Affective characteristics such as anxiety level, stability, dominance, or dependence influence physician-patient relationships and the degree of patient compliance with therapy. Health outcomes may therefore be affected not only by how well the physician manages the resulting problems but by how well he perceives and handles the underlying personality characteristics (Francis, Korsch, and Morris, 1969). Also, patients may range from those aware of the slightest body reaction to those who are almost oblivious of body reactions and their potential significance. Both extremes hamper effective and efficient medical care. The hypochondriac, in addition to overutilizing medical services, may miss serious problems even while seeking help for an imaginary problem. On the other hand, those who avoid identifying or acknowledging their symptoms, in addition to increasing the risk of missed diagnoses, may not seek help until too late in the natural history of the disease.

Among cognitive patient characteristics related to medical care and its assessment, the patient's intelligence, the accuracy and adequacy of health information, and the individual's problem-solving ability can all have an important influence on the perception of health and illness and the use of health services. Behavioral characteristics largely overlap with socioeconomic variables and lifestyle. Patient awareness of symptoms is often associated with socioeconomic or cultural background (Mechanic, 1968; Freidson, 1961). The ability to identify appropriate medical care facilities is necessary for the patient to obtain adequate care. A great deal is required of the patient to utilize available medical care resources well; there does not seem to be a satisfactory mechanism, for instance, for educating patients as to what facilities provide primary care for what problems. Lack of such information can be a deterrent to an optimal prognosis and a satisfactory health outcome.

Patients themselves must attain certain skills in obtaining adequate and appropriate care. This begins with learning when and when not to seek care and continues through followup for each problem. Relatively simple measures of such skills can be developed to assess these outcomes. Finally, patient compliance is a major health behavioral characteristic affecting outcomes. It depends on the patients' understanding of their role in therapy. Cooperation in following instructions given by the physician is essential, and patient education about prognosis and the effects of treatment as influenced by compliance may have a strong effect on health outcomes. This may include taking medication at the prescribed dosages and times, changing diet and physical activity habits, following special treatment, and returning for special diagnostic tests and followup appointments. Many patients are careless about taking pills; more than a third may skip them altogether or not complete the prescribed course of medication (Bergman and Werner, 1963). The reasons for noncompliance may be that the physician forgot to give proper instructions or that patients did not hear, understand, or remember the instructions given or decided that the possible benefits were not worth the disruption of their routine. Many behavior patterns, such as smoking, involve more complex determinants; noncompliance here may not be as amenable to casual physician influence. Each area is different, and potential for improvement through altered care must be determined carefully.

Exogenous Patient Factors
External or exogenous patient factors related to health and medical care include the physical environment, family, community and social groups, and local medical resources.

The physical environment of the patient, his occupation or other activities, or exposure to toxic substances, smog, or crowded living conditions are examples of relevant aspects. Factors of climate, such as extreme cold or humidity, may also affect patient health. Biological factors such as food sources and the common diseases of specific geographical areas often constitute hazards to health. If epidemiological data about such hazards exist, they can provide criteria for assessing both physician and patient education outcomes, as well as the efficiency of resource allocation.

The mechanisms of social control are equally relevant to health, although more difficult to assess or improve. Within the community, the family is probably a major source of the individual's attitudes toward health problems and health care. It may well be that quality of care assessment should focus on the medical care pattern of the whole family. An understanding of family stability and interaction might explain patient utilization patterns and put organic symptoms and complaints in better perspective.

Secondary social groups such as relatives, peer groups, and possibly neighborhood or occupational groups may affect health outcomes in indirect ways, since there is often a pooling of information, referrals to medical professionals or pseudoprofessionals, and even a sharing of medication. Also, formal organizations such as corporations, government, and schools influence individual and population health. They may directly promote broad preventive medicine, safety, and health education programs, and many organizations provide their own medical care facilities, such as factory health services or school health nurses.

The type of facility at which the patient receives care may be determined by financial status, insurance coverage, the organization of medical care in the area of residence, and the availability of transportation. Such exogenous patient characteristics may determine whether a patient will be treated by specialists in clinics or by medical students and house staff in university or county hospitals. The facilities available to the patient have a bearing on prognosis and health outcomes; and the use of resources and the awareness of health problem sources can and should provide the focus of assessment of the effectiveness and efficiency of community and outreach programs.

The Well Patient

Perhaps one of the greatest challenges to quality assurance are those aspects of health care relating to well patients. Here, problems of lifestyle, prevention, and health education may well have the greatest potential for health maintenance and improvement. In terms of numbers and of healthy life years to be gained, the group of well patients is of paramount importance for modern health care, but the health benefit potential encompassed by this group is usually not even recognized. Self-imposed risks have been shown to be significantly involved in the leading causes of morbidity and loss of life years (Lalonde, 1974). Smoking, drinking while driving, not using seatbelts, inappropriate diet, lack of exercise, inability to manage emotional stress from everyday living; overdependence on drugs to perk up, to sleep, to manage tension; sexual inadequacy and malfunction; nonawareness of or inability to maintain social support systems; inability to cope with isolation and depression; and inadequate parenting and the lack of socialization of new generations of children are among the many problems that may turn the well patient into a sick patient and cause preventable impairment.

There is mounting evidence that such problems can be successfully managed if people can be made aware of and given access to effective resources. Controlled community trials such as the Stanford Cardiovascular Study have documented substantial reduction of risk by educational means. Informed self-help, meditation, and procedures such as the use of life-stress scales are the object of much research and seem to have some value (Kristein, Arnold, and Wynder, 1977; Benson, 1975; Wyler, Masuda, and Holmes, 1971).

Quality assurance focus on management of the well patient would thus seem to offer potential in the future. As we become increasingly pessimistic about the net population benefits of traditional medicine, perhaps there is reason to be optimistic about the benefits to be realized in the largely uncharted waters of this field of preventive medicine.

THE HEALTH PROBLEM

In defining health problems, it is common to limit assessment to the small group composed of organic medical conditions. This in turn limits the assessment of the quality of health care to areas that may well not encompass substantial health benefit not achieved by current management, a concept discussed in detail in Chapter 3. The range of health factors outlined in the following should indicate topics for more comprehensive and effective quality assurance planning.

Patient and Physician Definitions
of Health Problems

An overview of the issues involved in who should define health problems has been provided by White (1973). At one extreme are those physician defined problems that have, or with sufficient research may have, recognized treatments or palliative measures. At the other extreme are those problems that are defined by patients and may or may not be related to known treatment effects. The physician's role is to help the patient better define and manage the problems of living more constructively and dying more comfortably without imposing intolerable burdens on oneself and others (White, 1973). Many of the problems currently presented to the medical profession are the problems of responses to the stresses and strains of domestic, occupational, and social life.

The most relevant application of this patient oriented approach to health care is in ambulatory practice. While hospital admitting problems are physician defined and readily codable by the International

Classification of Diseases, patients come to physicians with complaints (I'm having trouble getting to sleep at night), symptoms (I have this pain in my stomach), problems (My child's temper tantrums are getting out of control), inquiries (Should I stop taking my pills if they make me nauseous?), requests (Could I get a refill of my medicine?), and pseudodiagnoses (My "asthma" is giving me trouble). Health problems in ambulatory care are thus largely patient defined and require a new symptom classification scheme, an example of which is the one developed by Meads and McLemore (1974), building on the work of previous investigators. Friedlob et al. (1976) have reviewed the numerous classification systems currently available and have compiled a comprehensive review and analysis of such systems.

In ambulatory practice, therefore, most visits will not result in a simple codable diagnosis specifying a cause and indicating treatment. According to the National Ambulatory Medical Care Study (1973), the largest single group of presenting problems (nearly 36.5 percent) are nonsymptomatic and involve routine checkups such as well child, well adult, and prenatal care (18.5 percent) and progress visits (18 percent). The second largest group complains about pain (16 percent), from head (2 percent) to lower extremity (3.7 percent), with coughs and colds coming third (5 percent). It is evident that assessing the outcomes of such patient defined problems will require a unique method of definition, scaling, and prognosis. Research data on the natural history and prognosis of organic medical disease problems are scarce enough, but the problem of developing assessment standards for care of such common ailments as cough, tension headache, or obscure leg pain has almost no support in the literature. No etiology is evident, no diagnosis can be made, and most treatment is palliative or of questionable efficacy. It is likely that consensus estimates by experienced physicians will prove both essential and indispensable in developing assessment measures and standards for these common ambulatory patient problems and the quality of care rendered.

The distinction between patient and physician defined problems will also determine whether diagnostic or therapeutic outcomes are to be assessed. The initial population at risk sampled for assessing diagnostic outcomes should have a common patient defined problem or chief complaint, so that both misdiagnoses and missed diagnoses can be defined and measured (see Chapter 3 for a discussion of these). For example, for a population at risk consisting of patients whose complaint is abdominal pain, followup might indicate that 10 percent had renal or ureteral pathology and that 90 percent had bowel problems. If diagnostic accuracy for renal disease is assessed only on the basis of patients diagnosed as having renal disease, misdiagnoses or false positives (i.e., inaccurate renal diagnoses) may be identified, but missed diagnoses or false negatives (i.e., renal problems erroneously diagnosed as bowel conditions) will be lost to assessment. On the other hand, assessment of therapeutic outcomes requires a group of patients with a common diagnosis to ensure the homogeneity of prognosis necessary for establishing health outcome standards. For example, assessment focus on all patients with abdominal pain could lead to difficulties in defining meaningful standards for eventual health outcomes, since this group may represent bowel conditions (appendicitis or cholecystitis) or renal conditions (cancers, infections, and stones).

Thus, patient defined and physician defined health problems, although conceptually different, are both essential in planning quality assessment. Each carries with it unique considerations that must be recognized so as to identify the greatest achievable benefit not being achieved in present practice.

Benefit Analysis of Health Problems

Another way of examining health problems for assessment and improvement potential would be their categorization by specific prognostic classes, correlating these with projected population health impairment in the absence of treatment. This could provide a tentative health benefit classification. However, although we know the microbial causes of infectious disease, the antecedent events of physical-chemical trauma, and the mismatch of many genetic characteristics that cause congenital defects, the primary causes of most psychiatric disorders, degenerative diseases, neoplasms, endocrine disorders, inflammatory diseases, and the myriad vague complaints managed in ambulatory practice are little understood. These conditions are rarely cured and often not adequately palliated because of our meager understanding of their etiology. On the other hand, that information that is available is usually sufficiently specific to permit expert consensus on the potential for health improvement and prevention of impairment by adequate medical management (Rutstein et al., 1976).

The major etiological groups in this proposed classification are related to theoretical prognostic potential and expected group impairment in Table 4.1. The somewhat arbitrarily constituted categories are arrayed on two axes, i.e., in order of decreasing health benefit, ranging from cure to palliation if care is provided; and in order of decreasing population impairment in the absence of formal

Table 4.1. Examples of health benefit analysis of major etiological categories of health problems

Projected Population Impairment if not Treated[a]	Prognosis if Treated				
	Amenable to complete prevention or cure	Partially amenable to prevention or cure	Amenable to substantial control	Amenable to partial control	Amenable to caring and palliation only
HIGH	Physical and chemical trauma	Nonbacterial and nonspirochetal infectious disease	Congenital visual problems, refraction, glaucoma	Early degenerative disease	
	Bacterial and spirochetal infectious disease	Conception and complications of pregnancy	Allergies: hayfever, asthma	Arthritis and rheumatic disorders	
			Bipolar depression	Mild to moderate psychiatric disorders: neuroses, psychophysiological problems,	
			Inadequate parenting: personality growth/development	personality disorders, delinquency, dependency, alcoholism	
			Recurrent idiopathic organ system disorders		
MODERATE	Nutrition disorders: over and under-nourishment— obesity, pernicious anemia, ricketts	Iatrogenic disorders: drug reactions, effects of unnecessary surgery, psychic effects of maleducation	Hypertension and congestive heart failure	Endocrine disorders	Severe mental and emotional disorders: psychoses, character disorders, organic brain syndromes
			Stress syndromes: occupational, marital, social, and personal	Learning disorders	Late degenerative disease
		Common visual problems	Discontent syndromes: dissatisfaction, loneliness, occupational boredom, geriatric maladjustment		Late or inaccessible neoplasms
LOW	Rare skin carcinoma	Congenital disorders	Fluid and electrolyte disorders	Metabolic disorders	

[a]Estimated as impairment per person that would occur if no care were provided times the number of patients involved in the population.

medical care. The health problems range from physical trauma and infectious diseases to learning disorders and stress syndromes, and both traditional medical-organic factors and more complex emotional and mental problems are included. Since any of these problems may require or receive medical attention, all should be considered when defining a topic with a view to achievable benefit not achieved (Emlet et al., 1971).

Health Problem Complications and Combinations

In planning outcome assessment, each important combination of health problems must usually be considered as a single entity for purposes of developing evaluation measures and standards. The addition of any major complication or disease that would substantially alter medical management or prognosis for a patient group usually requires reformulation of assessment measures and standards. Prevalence factors are obvious serious constraints in assessing such problems.

In weighing one health problem against another for potential outcome assessment, therefore, the likelihood, severity, and manageability of complications either of the health problem itself, such as pulmonary emboli from lower leg thrombophlebitis, or of an associated therapy, such as iatrogenic hemorrhage from use of anticoagulants, must be considered. Complications may be worse than the disease itself (meningitis complicating otitis media in children) or little more than a nuisance (laryngitis complicating pharyngitis). The efficacy of interventions in preventing or managing complications is the key factor in weighing prognostic significance and improvement potential.

Another important consideration is the presence of multiple health problems, although only one will generally be the primary reason for contact with health care personnel. Combinations also vary in prognostic implications, some having a worse prognosis and some a better prognosis than the sum of all problems separately. Examples of important and often neglected diagnostic combinations that illustrate meaningful topics of care assessment are gall bladder disease combined with upper gastrointestinal problems such as ulcers or hiatus hernias, hemorrhoids and colonic polyps, appendicitis and pelvic inflammatory disease, diabetes and heart failure, coronary insufficiency or occlusion and acute or subacute surgical problems, severe arthritis and peptic ulcers, and left ventricular failure and emphysema. Multiple health problems are also frequent in chronic disease or impairment, where both combinations and complications of health problems may compound the problems of prognosis and assessment of care.

Development of outcome standards thus must take into account the characteristics of each condition, and assessment of priorities will require the clustering of patients according to the more prevalent and important group of diseases that they have in common.

THE PROVIDERS OF CARE

The third element in the health care process, the providers, operate within a complex health care delivery structure. At the individual medical practice level, structural shortcomings of the health care system may seem to be outside the traditional mandate of quality assurance and should be addressed at the political level. However, a community's treatment facilities and equipment and its personnel as well as its resources can provide a meaningful focus for group quality assurance efforts, in particular with regard to identifying correctable determinants of seriously deficient outcomes of care.

Health Care Personnel

Among the complex hierarchy of services and professional medical personnel involved in the provision of care, three levels can be usefully identified for quality assurance planning: primary, secondary, and tertiary care. Primary care professionals provide first contact care and usually assume comprehensive, continuous, and long-term responsibility for patient health needs. Primary care physicians would therefore seem to be an especially meaningful focus for health outcome studies. This group consists of general or family practitioners, pediatricians, general internists, general dentists, and occasionally, general surgeons and possibly obstetricians and gynecologists. However, although the potential for realizing achievable benefits of care is in all likelihood considerable in ambulatory primary practice, quality assurance in this field faces a range of theoretical and practical problems that render both the establishment of valid assessment standards and the measurement of care deficiencies extremely difficult. It is well recognized that, especially in solo practice, the type of illnesses presented to primary care physicians, problems of record keeping and data collection for assessment studies, and constraints of time and funds have all delayed development of effective quality assurance strategies in ambulatory care (Palmer, 1976).

Secondary and tertiary care, in large part based on referral from primary care physicians, is provided by specialists who focus on organ systems, such as cardiologists, urologists, or ophthalmologists; or on tissues and cells, such as pathologists or oncologists. The care they provide is often at a more complex technical level, limited in scope and time, and frequently rendered in the hospital or at medical centers. Initial outcome assessment of care by these provider groups, although important, may contain less potential for large-scale population benefit than assessing care rendered by primary care physicians. However, the general principles of outcome assessment and improvement, albeit more limited in content and scope, apply also to specific health problems such as late stage kidney failure, rehabilitation of paraplegics, metastatic carcinoma, endarterectomy, coronary bypass surgery, or corneal transplants.

The outcome approach to quality assurance is also valuable for the assessment of care by other health professionals such as nurses, pharmacists, dieticians, and laboratory technicians. In terms of numbers alone, nurses make up the largest single group of health care providers. Since they usually implement a management plan developed by the physician in addition to their own management, the specific effects of nursing care will have to be studied from a somewhat different point of view. On the other hand, assessment of nursing care is an important aspect of secondary studies conducted to identify determinants of established deficiencies of care. Also, this group of health care personnel is a useful focus for initial assessment of care interaction outcomes in those diagnostic and therapeutic processes for which they are solely responsible. Another significant outcome assessment aspect of nursing is that of educational outcomes, in which the nurse's or therapist's success in facilitating patient learning is extremely important and can be readily assessed. Also, health professionals at this level have much to contribute to the setting of priorities in general, and particularly in those problem areas where their experience may provide special insights. They have much to offer in prognostic judgment based on their more detailed and frequent patient contacts.

Although pharmacists are officially in a supporting role, they may actually provide a form of primary care for a large number of people who seek over the counter recommendations. This aspect could furnish material for some interesting health outcome studies. Efficiency measures of the extent to which pharmacists cooperate with physicians to facilitate generic prescribing or help the patient obtain the highest quality drug at the lowest price might be of interest. At the present time, traditional accreditation mechanisms are used to assure the competence of pharmacists. Equally valuable might be recognition of the innovative new career roles of pharmacists as central therapeutic coordinators and analysts. Due to the present preponderance of specialty as opposed to general medicine, the pharmacist is often the only central point for prescriptions from many physicians for the same patient. Monitoring for duplication or antagonistic combinations might be an important task for the pharmacist and might be well worth assessment of achievable benefits not achieved in this field.

Managers and administrators should be the focus of efficiency studies to identify areas where cost might be reduced or administrative and resource management improved. This type of personnel can and should apply the results of cost-benefit studies to their own organizations and contribute to assessment priority decisions and to specific quality assessment studies with a utilization or economic component.

Physical Resources and Facilities

Modern health care depends to a great extent upon medical and related technology. If specialized equipment is not available, if supplies are missing, or if records are inadequate, the quality of medical care may well suffer. On the other hand, the presence of such resources does not necessarily indicate their adequate use. Here, the problem for assessment of care lies in identifying those resources that are crucial to effective and efficient care of the predominant problems presented by a given population. Existing and accepted standards for assessment of health care structure are valuable and should be integrated with overall quality assurance functions; the measurement of structural characteristics (i.e., structural outcomes) has provided the most widespread assessment approach in the health field. Unfortunately, there is often little basis for inferring adequate health outcomes even if structure is acceptable. Consequently, these variables might well be analyzed to identify correctable determinants of deficient health outcomes or care processes.

Clinics and Hospitals. For hospitals and group practice clinics, accreditation bodies check such structural aspects as buildings, furniture, equipment, and records. Specific accreditation standards are published for a wide variety of medical care facilities (Donabedian, 1969). Traditional quality assessment methods for hospitals have included facility measures developed by the Joint Commission on Accreditation of Hospitals (1971); for group practice clinics, measures developed by the American Group Practice Association have been used. These methods have been expanded and now include assessment of a variety of other outcomes, including diagnostic and patient health aspects (Jacobs, Christoffel, and Dixon, 1976).

The contents of the practitioner's office, including its supplies and the equipment needed for medical practice, have been listed by more than one group interested in developing accreditation mechanisms (Commission on Accreditation, 1972; Commission on Child Health Care, 1972). While office facilities alone are likely to be a poor indicator of the quality of medical care, they can be used to help define correctable determinants of deficient health outcomes. A pediatric practice that has neither an incubator nor a nearby bacteriology laboratory might explain failure to diagnose and treat Group A beta hemolytic streptococcal pharyngitis.

Hospitals and their outpatient facilities are among the most vital community resources for medical care; they are also among those most relevant to structural outcome assessment. Management of acute myocardial infarction suspects in elaborate coronary care units can provide a dramatic focus for quality assessment. However, the majority of patients usually do not require such elaborate technological support. An uncomplicated pregnancy patient in labor is one of the most frequent admissions to a short stay hospital, and common surgical procedures such as tonsillectomy, appendectomy, cholecystectomy, and hysterectomy account for a large proportion of surgical admissions. For these cases, even modestly equipped hospitals offer much scope for assessment of health outcomes. Here, it may be more important to assess misuse of resources than lack of sophisticated equipment. The hospital's potential for harm, through drug errors or toxicity effects, infections resistant to antibiotics, or the psychic trauma that frequently lasts long after hospital discharge must be considered. For example, it has been shown that a percentage of patients misdiagnosed as having myocardial infarction may become unnecessary cardiac cripples after several weeks in a coronary care unit (Cassem and Hackett, 1971). Negative effects that detract from the net value of care should be an area of special quality assurance attention.

Hospital emergency rooms are growing in number and utilization and provide a source of primary care for many serious acute and chronic illnesses. However, studies have indicated that only one-third of emergency room patients have a clear medical emergency, that another one-third have conditions that are not clinically confirmed emergencies, and that the final third use the emergency room chiefly as a source of convenient primary care (Weinerman et al., 1966). Nonetheless, the availability of good emergency care facilities, with a range of subspecialties on call, can make a considerable difference to health outcomes in a limited number of problems, especially in surgery. Because outcomes are often determined in a short time span and because records are available for sampling patients with a given problem, the emergency room could be an excellent location for both diagnostic and therapeutic outcome assessment (Kaszuba and Gibson, 1978; Sadler, Sadler, and Webb, 1977; Gibson, 1976; Brook, Berg, and Schechter, 1973).

As a rule, in studies of diagnostic outcomes, only misdiagnoses can be determined from hospital data. The physician's office is the principal locus of original diagnoses and referrals for hospital admission; this is where missed diagnoses will have to be found (Donabedian, 1969). Also, only provisional outcomes can be assessed in the hospital. Conclusive outcome determination nearly always requires patient observation weeks, months, or even years after discharge. Thus, the period of hospitalization by itself provides a rather narrow focus for conclusive health outcome assessment. Yet it can provide an exceptional resource for patient surveys and subsequent outpatient followup because of the availability of discharge abstracts for sampling (as opposed to assessment) purposes.

Long-term Care Facilities. Facilities and services providing long-term care are an increasingly important and expensive component of health services. The problems posed by this sector in terms of resources, their allocation, and their use and the emphasis on maintenance, functional rehabilitation, and psychosocial aspects of care are reflected in the growth of data and information indicating a wide range of needs, deficiencies, and requirements. Quality assurance can and must make important contributions to the assessment and improvement of outcomes in this area. Data reported by the National Center for Health Statistics show that the long-term institutional population of all ages has grown from 1.6 million in 1963 to nearly 2 million in 1969 (Sherwood, 1975). The proportion of the mentally or physically handicapped or chronically ill aged in institutions is over one million, and a large number of these are affected not only by physical ailments and impairments but also by emotional problems, mental disorders, and chronic brain syndromes (Stotsky, 1970).

There has been increasingly vocal criticism of many aspects of institutional long-term care, whether in nursing homes, in facilities for the mentally ill or retarded, or in other types of institutions. Also, there is now growing emphasis on practical and presumably less costly alternatives encompassed by home care services, such as sheltered housing, home nursing, and homemaker services to name only a few (Senate Special Committee on Aging, 1971). However, there is little hard evidence at the moment of the generally greater effectiveness of noninstitutional over institutional care or of the specific populations who might derive greater benefit from one or the other alternative. In view of the multiple health problems often affecting the chronically ill (whether physically or mentally), an outcome approach focusing on functional status should offer considerable potential for improving the effectiveness and efficiency of care, both in terms of individual patient health and of resource allocation.

Another major issue in long-term care is the identification of target populations, taking into consideration that long-term care encompasses the entire spectrum of caring and curing efforts and requires a broad range of health professionals, ranging from physicians and nurses to physiotherapists and psychological counselors. It is generally accepted that long-term care should provide both therapeutic and rehabilitative management to restore levels of function or to maintain present levels of functioning and to prevent or defer further deterioration, in addition to supportive care during the terminal stage of life (Sherwood, 1975). This implies the need for reliable and valid tools for assessing the functional, social, and psychological status of patients as well as their needs and improvement potential. Such measures, although plentiful, are still very far from being generally applicable or accepted, and their development remains a crucial issue, particularly with regard to the quality of the patient's life as distinct from measures of appropriate placement, assignment of nursing care, and similar aspects of medical management of isolated health problems.

Medical Records. Medical records are of great importance in any assessment of care, and themselves constitute an area of substantial improvement potential. Their exact relationship to health outcomes remains open, but some studies have indicated a correlation between poor records and poor care (Payne and Lyons, 1972; Clute, 1963; Trussell, Morehead, and Ehrlich, 1962; Peterson et al., 1956; Rosenfeld, 1957).

Patient records in ambulatory medical care are of first concern. The fact that most office records are of poor quality has been documented (Tenney, White, and Williamson, 1974). In a pilot study for the National Ambulatory Medical Care Survey, a national sampling of physicians was to yield record data that would provide a profile of the care given by ambulatory care physicians. However, nearly one physician in five had no record other than the name and charge; roughly two in five had such incomplete recording of data that patient complaints, diagnoses, and treatments could not be tabulated. Less than one in five had records meeting even the minimum standards of the survey. Because of these findings, record review was abandoned as a procedural approach to that study. The inadequacy of office records for medical audit has also been confirmed (Osborne and Thompson, 1975).

Among the more recent efforts to develop a uniform data base for ambulatory care medical office records is the ambulatory care encounter data set (Murnaghan, 1973), which suggests fifteen information categories, including demographic data, patient attributes, and service and administration elements. Unfortunately, outcome data based on followup will probably not be included. The most important use of present ambulatory care chart data for quality assurance is in permitting development of a sample frame, which is a tabulation of all patients having the characteristics qualifying them for study. From this list, a smaller sample can be identified and followed prospectively for outcome assessment. If records are not sufficiently complete to develop a sample frame, other methods can be used, such as those developed in the author's health accounting system (see Chapters 6-10).

Hospital records are of greater utility for quality assurance, but here, too, much remains to be done. The efforts of the Joint Commission on Accreditation of Hospitals have resulted in a general upgrading of the quality of patient records. Since the early 1950s, nearly 2,000 hospitals in the United States, Canada, and several other countries have adopted the uniform hospital abstract system developed under the auspices of the Commission on Professional and Hospital Activities. The data generated by the Professional Activity Study (PAS) have facilitated traditional utilization review and medical audit studies. Also, a hospital discharge abstract set has been developed with a view to establishing a common information base for hospital discharge data based on standard definitions, classifications, and measurement methods (Murnaghan and White, 1970). However, the forms proposed and utilized under these and various other regional information systems still offer only a limited basis for outcome assessment.

Despite progress in the field, many hospital chart data are still insufficient even for process review. In a study of performance in twenty-two nonfederal short-term hospitals in Hawaii, Payne and Lyons (1972) found that about one in three of a basic list of important performance variables was not recorded on the hospital charts. The major shortcomings of hospital records for evaluation of either processes or outcomes can be summarized as follows:

- No check is possible on the quality of recorded data;
- A substantial percentage of relevant hospital data are not recorded;
- Pertinent preadmission ambulatory care data are often not recorded;
- Focus on organic pathology often precludes recording of psychosocial factors, patient understanding, and compliance information;
- Missed diagnoses go unrecognized, especially for patients who are not admitted and thus have no charts;
- Health outcomes are usually not recorded except as "improved," "not improved," or "worse" at discharge; and
- Postdischarge followup data are not obtained.

Nonetheless, hospital records remain a valuable resource in that they provide an exceptional base for case sampling for a given health problem, allow verification of recorded diagnoses from recorded data as well as identification of some missed diagnoses by routine screening test data, and permit the establishment of provisional outcomes before discharge, such as fracture healing or a live infant from a successful delivery. Both hospital and office records, therefore, are an important assessment resource, and their improvement should be a major goal of health care in the future. Here, it is important to recognize that a successful quality assurance system cannot be limited by either the content or the completeness of existing patient record systems. The use of prospective assessment strategies and of carefully designed encounter forms will be crucial in the future.

Pharmaceuticals, Medical Supplies, and Equipment. Medicines, whether prescribed or nonprescribed, are among the most widely used resources in contemporary health care, and pharmaceutical substances and appliances constitute a substantial portion of medical care expenditures (Goddard, 1973). The implications for assessing both the efficiency and effectiveness of the use of these resources are obvious. Pharmaceutical preparations are especially good topics because of easily accessible consensual data on efficacy gathered by Food and Drug Administration teams (White, 1974). Prescription practices for any provider group should be monitored and the results compared to known standards of acceptability in terms of beneficial and detrimental patient effects. However, conflicting reports on the safety and efficacy of new drugs, the strong commercial pressures in the marketplace, and the wide range of hazards, side effects, contra-indications, and precautions demand careful, objective, and expert team judgment for interpretation. Gradually, an increasing number of products are being subjected to thorough and systematic scrutiny. As a matter of prudence, the results of this effort should be utilized in quality assessment, as well as in medical practice in general.

Unfortunately, required proof of safety and efficacy of devices, equipment, and supplies is still largely unregulated, though this is now the responsibility of the Food and Drug Administration. Effective regulatory mechanisms are still lacking, and the provider must assume the responsibility of assuring the patient of established benefit and safety.

Medical Communication and Transportation. Physicians provide substantial diagnostic and therapeutic patient management over the telephone, especially outside of office hours. Telephone communication is also an increasingly important tool for the accurate evaluation and emergency care of poison or accident victims, the suicidal, and patients with acute abdominal and chest pain. Telephone counselors require both diagnostic and therapeutic expertise; they must also be skilled in achieving patient understanding and in eliciting compliance within minutes under the stress of an emergency situation. Telephone triage of medical emergencies is an especially relevant focus for quality assurance. In Russia, for instance, physicians who are specialists in emergency medicine supervise the handling of emergency medical telephone calls (Storey and Roth, 1971); in this country physicians are rarely trained in triage or emergency management by telephone, and considerable health loss may well result from the use of unqualified personnel.

The performance of medical transportation facilities is equally important. For instance, in myocardial infarction or acute trauma, swift transportation can mean the difference between life and death (Pell and D'Alonzo, 1964). Again, the Soviet Union has an extensively developed medical emergency system in which specialized ambulances are run by physicians and assistants; these are dispatched by a medical specialist from a central emergency switchboard (Storey and Roth, 1971; Fry, 1969). In the past few years many cities of the United States (e.g., Baltimore, Chicago, Minneapolis, San Diego, and Seattle) have been improving these services with the help of federal subsidies. The precise effect of such transportation deficiencies is unknown; it should be carefully considered in outcome assessment, especially for emergency health problems.

Practice Settings and Financing Mechanisms

The organization and financing of health care has a profound influence on both focus and motivation of quality assurance activities. The traditional organization of services, based on fee for service home, office, and hospital care, has become much more complex, with emphasis on progressive patient care and a proliferation of different institutions, financing sources, and payment methods (Breslow, 1974; Hepner and Hepner, 1973; Donabedian, 1973). While the predominant mode of health care delivery in the United States is still based on the solo practitioner's office, group practice has had a slow but steady growth (National Center for Health Statistics, 1975), and providing quality care at lower cost may have a competitive advantage (Saward, 1973). Nearly 80 percent of all physician-patient contacts are in an ambulatory setting, though this is down 10 percent from the midfifties, when over 90 percent of physician contacts were in an outpatient setting (Knowles, 1973).

However, as mentioned before, both group and solo practice models for quality assessment in ambulatory care pose a number of problems (Greene, 1976; Shapiro et al., 1976). Some group practice assessment results will be shown in Chapters 8-10. Few systems of quality assurance have been tried in solo practice, and its potential value in this setting is only inferred. The major practical problems are standards development, finding adequate numbers of patients with a given problem to warrant assessment effort, and the small but necessary amount of physician consultation time with quality assurance personnel. A possible approach might involve the organization of several solo practitioners in a joint quality assurance consortium. By pooling their patients for sampling purposes, the problem of numbers might be solved. The group could meet several times a year, once for setting priorities and several times for designing two or three studies that could be implemented with the help of assistant personnel, such as the health accountant in the author's quality assurance system (see Chapter 6). The documentation of effectiveness in health maintenance for the patient groups studied and the specific focus for continuing education efforts where improvement proves necessary could make such an experience meaningful to solo practitioners as well.

The affiliation of community hospitals or clinics with university teaching hospitals, on the other hand, provides an organizational setting that offers many advantages for quality of care assessment. In university practice, there is often a general pride in keeping up with current knowledge and maintaining high standards, and there also is a manpower supply of interns and residents who may be interested in assessment aspects. The university hospital offers a ready pool of subspecialty experts for priority and assessment criteria development. The drawback here is that an elitist attitude may tend to hamper quality assurance activity. University medical staff often feel that they set the highest standards for medical practice in the community and so are above quality assessment and the effort required in this respect. What they too often overlook is that their expertise frequently has a narrow focus on relatively uncommon organic medical conditions, and there is ground to question the quality of care and of caring rendered in university centers for the more common ailments (Payne et al., 1976; Rhee, 1975).

Furthermore, outcome assessment methods may be profoundly influenced by the method of provider payment, whether fee for service or prepaid. Fee for service payments, whether directly by the patient, by third party payors such as commercial insurance companies or Blue Cross/Blue Shield, or by foundations, account for the large majority of the care presently provided in this country (Andreopoulos, 1972). Physicians working on a fee for service basis only rarely provide care to an enrolled population. It has been charged that fee for service practice encourages a measurable, albeit unconscious, tendency toward overutilization, including return office visits and hospitalizations (Bellin and Kavaler, 1971). Curative services, as opposed to preventive services and early screening, are stressed. The bias induced by this type of payment plan is reflected in diagnostic outcomes, especially unwarranted positive diagnoses. Diagnostic and therapeutic evaluation might well focus on the "unnecessaries," such as unneeded laboratory tests, drugs, hospitalization or surgery, excessive mutual referrals, and unneeded x-rays (Bellin and Kavaler, 1971; Senate Committee on Finance, 1970). Unfortunately, the motives underlying these problems also make it likely that the use of "productive time" for quality assurance purposes will be considered wasteful.

Prepaid medical care plans still account for less than a fifth of patient visits. In a prepaid plan, a yearly fee may be paid by the individual member, jointly by the employee and the employer, or wholly by the government. The plan is then responsible for the health care of its subscribers or enrollees; most expenses are assumed. Here, the bias of concern is that of underutilization, as physicians may profit directly if overall costs are kept within a certain minimum for the group as a whole. On the other hand, total care is provided to an enrolled population so that continuity of care is more likely, and preventive and early detection services may be stressed. Administrative accounting also requires and provides fairly good patient records, as well as incentives for quality assurance activity. In this context, outcome assessment might focus on diagnostic outcomes, especially missed diagnoses, and on late stage disease. Another major factor in financing is the relative proportion of direct and indirect payments, which include private insurance and public payments. The steady drop of direct payments and the increase in insurance and public financing of care is well known. The implications of the change in payment source are for efficiency more than for effectiveness assessment. In a summary of the findings from his economic studies, Feldstein (1973) showed the rise in hospital costs to be mainly the result of the increased use of indirect payment sources. He states that because net out of pocket cost appears so modest, the patient is willing to buy more frequent and expensive care than he would if he were not insured. This fact, together with a rapid increase in consumer demand for sophisticated hospital services, has also been stressed by Knowles (1973). Provider willingness to keep up with this demand has resulted in a change in patient day cost from $16 in 1950 to $103 in 1972, while out of pocket expense has risen only from $10 to $19, correcting for dollar devaluation (Feldstein, 1973).

The implications of these findings for quality assurance are evident. For example, a fivefold increase in hospital laboratory costs (Knowles, 1973) should lead us to reconsider the use of multiple laboratory examinations, particularly where available treatments of abnormalities found may make little difference. Even a limited efficiency assessment study consisting of a literature search on the cost effectiveness of expensive equipment, based on explicit standards of acceptable error tolerance, would seem worthwhile. On the other hand, an example of underutilization is the failure to treat debilitating illness in nursing homes, where physicians are under the capitation method of reimbursement, so as to reduce costs (Bellin and Kavaler, 1971).

SUMMARY

An understanding of the wide range of health care content factors is important for quality assurance planning. Innovative combinations of patient, health problem, and provider characteristics are needed to determine the most valuable topics for assessment. There are many individual variables that affect the health of the patient and how he deals with health problems. These variables include endogenous factors such as age, sex, heredity, and behavior, and exogenous factors such as social and occupational environment and the availability and accessibility of health care resources. Many of these factors must be considered for an improvement of health outcomes.

A broad classification of health problems beyond the traditional group of organic medical conditions is also essential for comprehensive quality assurance planning. Patient defined problems, the most frequent problems in ambulatory practice, must be recognized in planning diagnostic outcome studies, while physician defined problems are most applicable to therapeutic studies. Health problems can also be classified etiologically according to theoretical cure or care potential and expected group impairment so as to facilitate setting assessment priorities. Further considerations for assessment planning are health problem complications and combinations.

The assessment content characteristics of the provider comprise personnel, facilities, and aspects of health care delivery such as practice settings and services. Primary care physicians and nurses are meaningful targets for outcome assessment, and assessment of specialists, therapists, administrators, and technicians at the secondary and tertiary levels of care can often be valuable. Assessment focusing on such provider characteristics as group or solo practice; fee for service or prepaid payment systems; clinic, hospital, or long-term care facilities; or on medical records and supporting services can indicate valuable areas for performance improvement.

Accessibility and availability of health care services have until recently depended more on local resources, on social factors and physical geography, and on private initiative than on established health care needs, as the poor and rural areas of this country demonstrate. Self-help, voluntarism, and local public involvement in medical care are esteemed. Emphasis has been on fragmented, episodic, crisis oriented acute care, with common chronic conditions considered uninteresting and preventive care neglected. Due in large part to such factors, health care is in a period of social and economic transition in which change, for better or worse, is being enforced by legislation. The goal is the achievement of more effective and efficient medical care (Hepner and Hepner, 1973). In the face of impending change, an understanding of the forces restructuring the health care system in this country may provide some of the most cogent reasons for the active personal involvement of providers of care in quality assurance programs. Constructive action may well modify the present potential for an overly regulated profession. Professional leadership in active, ongoing quality assurance systems can produce consistent and substantial, documented improvement in the attainment of achievable health benefits not being achieved at present. Enough prototypes are now available and enough health services research studies have been published to support systematic approaches to direct assessment and improvement.

REFERENCES

Andreopoulos, S., 1972. Medical cure and medical care—the organization and financing of personal health care services. *Milbank Mem Fund Q* 50(4) pt. 2:225-38.

Bellin, L.E., and Kavaler, F. 1971. Medicaid practitioner abuses and excuses vs counterstrategy of the New York City Health Department. *Am J Public Health* 62:2201-10.

Benson, H. 1975. *The Relaxation Response.* New York: Morrow.

Bergman, A.B., and Werner, R.J. 1963. Failure of children to receive penicillin by mouth. *N Engl J Med* 268:1334-38.

Breslow, L. 1974. Quality and cost control: Medicare and beyond. *Med Care* 12:95-114.

Brook, R.H.; Berg, M.H.; and Schechter, P.A. 1973. Effectiveness of nonemergency care via an emergency room—a study of 116 patients with gastrointestinal symptoms. *Ann Intern Med* 78:333-39.

Cassem, N.H., and Hackett, T.P. 1971. Psychiatric consultation in a coronary care unit. *Ann Intern Med* 75:9-14.

Clute, K.F. 1963. *The General Practitioner—A Study of Medical Education and Practice in Ontario and Nova Scotia.* Toronto: University of Toronto Press.

Commission on Accreditation. 1972. *Accreditation Protocol of the American Association of Medical Clinics.* Alexandria, Va.: American Association of Medical Clinics.

Commission on Child Health Care. 1972. *Standards of Child Health Care.* 2nd ed. Evanstown, Ill.: American Academy of Pediatrics.

Donabedian, A. 1969. *A Guide to Medical Care Administration.* Vol 2: *Medical Care Appraisal—Quality and Utilization.* New York: American Public Health Association.

———. 1973. *Aspects of Medical Care Administration: Specifying Requirements for Health Care.* Cambridge: Harvard University Press.

Emlet, H.E.; Williamson, J.W.; Casey, I.; and Davis, J.L. 1971. *Alternative Methods for Estimating Health Care Benefits and Required Resources.* Vol. 1: *Summary.* Falls Church, Va.: Analytic Services.

Feldstein, M.S. 1973. The medical economy. *Sci Am* 229(3):151-66.

Francis, V.; Korsch, B.M.; and Morris, M.J. 1969. Gaps in doctor-patient communication—patient's response to medical advice. *N Engl J Med* 280: 535-40.

Fraser, F.C. 1973. Genetic counseling. In *Medical Genetics*, V.A. McKusick and R. Claiborne, eds., pp. 221-28. New York: HP Publishing.

Freidson, E. 1961. *Patient's Views of Medical Practice: A Study of Subscribers to a Prepaid Medical Plan in the Bronx.* New York: Russell Sage Foundation.

Friedlob, A.; Caro, D.; Shimitz, R.; McClain, M.; O'Connor, J.P.; and Batalden, P. 1976. *A Review of Medical Care Classification Systems for Use in Ambulatory Care.* Minneapolis: St. Louis Park Medical Center Research Foundation.

Fry, J. 1969. *Medicine in Three Societies—A Comparison of Medical Care in the USSR, USA, and UK.* New York: American Elsevier.

Gibson, G. 1976. EMS evaluation: criteria for standards and research design. *Health Serv Res* 11:105-11.

Goddard, J.L. 1973. The medical business. *Sci Am* 229(3):161-66.

Greene, R. 1976. *Assuring Quality in Medical Care: The State of the Art.* Cambridge, Mass.: Ballinger.

Hepner, J.O., and Hepner, D.M. 1973. *The Health Strategy Game: A Challenge for Reorganization and Management.* St. Louis: Mosby.

Jacobs, C.M.; Christoffel, T.H.; and Dixon, W. 1976. *Measuring the Quality of Patient Care—The Rationale for Outcome Audit.* Cambridge, Mass.: Ballinger.

Joint Commission on Accreditation of Hospitals. 1971. *Accreditation Manual for Hospitals: Hospital Accreditation Program.* Chicago: Joint Commission on Accreditation of Hospitals.

Kaszuba, N.L., and Gibson, G. 1978. Severity, satisfaction and symptom resolution in patients of emergency medicine residents. *J Am Coll Emerg Physicians* 7:192-97.

Knowles, J.H. 1973. The hospital. *Sci Am* 229(3):128-37.

Kristein, M.M.; Arnold, C.B.; and Wynder, E.L. 1977. Health economics and preventive care. *Science* 195:457-62.

Lalonde, M. 1974. *A New Perspective on the Health of Canadians.* Government of Canada, Ottawa.

Lerner, M. 1977. The non-health services determinants of health levels: conceptualization and public policy recommendations. In *Issues in Promoting Health,* Committee Reports of the Medical Sociology Section of the American Sociological Association. *Med Care* 15(5)supplement:74-83.

Meads, S., and McLemore, T. 1974. The national ambulatory medical care survey—symptom classification. *Vital Health Stat* 2(63):1-35.

Mechanic, D. 1968. *Medical Sociology: A Selective View.* New York: The Free Press.

Murnaghan, J.H., ed. 1973. *Ambulatory Medical Care Data. Report of the Conference on Ambulatory Care Records.* Philadelphia: Lippincott. Reprinted from *Med Care* 11(2)supplement.

Murnaghan, J.H., and White, K.L., eds. 1970. *Hospital Discharge Data. Report of the Conference on Hospital Discharge Abstracts Systems.* Philadelphia: Lippincott. Reprinted from *Med Care* 8(4)supplement.

National Ambulatory Medical Care Study. 1973. Pilot test data analyzed by students at The Johns Hopkins University School of Hygiene and Public Health. Baltimore: Department of Medical Care and Hospitals (processed).

National Center for Health Statistics. 1975. *The National Ambulatory Medical Care Survey: 1973 Summary. United States, May 1973-April 1974.* Vital and Health Statistics, Series 13, No. 21. Rockville, Md.: Department of Health Education and Welfare, Publication No. (HRA) 76-1772.

Osborne, C.E., and Thompson, H.C. 1975. Criteria for evaluation of ambulatory child health care by chart audit. Development and testing of a methodology. *Pediatrics* 56(4) pt. 2:625-92.

Palmer, R.H. 1976. Choice of strategies. In *Assuring Quality in Medical Care,* R. Greene, ed., ch. 3. Cambridge, Mass.: Ballinger.

Payne, B.C.; Lyons, T.F.; Dwarshins, L.; Kolton, M.; and Morris, W. 1976. *Quality of Medical Care: Evaluation and Improvement.* Health Services Monograph Series T40. Chicago: Hospital Research and Education Trust.

Payne, B.C., and Lyons, T.F. 1972. *Method of Evaluating and Improving Personal Medical Care Quality—Episode of Illness Study for Hawaii Medical Association.* Ann Arbor: University of Michigan School of Medicine.

Pell, S., and D'Alonzo, C.A. 1964. Immediate mortality and five year survival of employed men with a first M.I. *N Engl J Med* 270:915-22.

Peterson, O.L.; Andrews, L.P.; Spain, R.S.; and Greenberg, B.G. 1956. An analytic study of North Carolina general practice, 1953-1954. *J Med Educ* 31(12) pt. 2.

Ranofsky, A.L. 1973. *Inpatient Utilization of Short-Stay Hospitals by Diagnosis: United States, 1968.* National Center for Health Statistics, Vital and Health Statistics, Series 13, No. 12. Rockville, Md.: Department of Health, Education and Welfare, Publication No. (HSM) 73-1763.

Rhee, S.O. 1975. Relative influence of specialty status, organization of office care and organization of hospital care on the quality of medical care—a multivariate analysis. Doctoral thesis, University of Michigan, Ann Arbor.

Rosenfeld, L.S. 1957. Quality of medical care in hospitals. *Am J Public Health* 47:856-65.

Rutstein, D.D.; Berenberg, W.; Chalmers, T.C.; Child, C.G.; Fishman, A.P.; and Perrin, E.B. 1976. Measuring the quality of medical care—a clinical method. *N Engl J Med* 294:582-88.

Sadler, A.M., Jr.; Sadler, B.L.; and Webb, S.B. 1977. *Emergency Medical Care—The Neglected Public Service.* Cambridge, Mass.: Ballinger.

Saward, E.W. 1973. The organization of medical care. *Sci Am* 229(3):169-75.

Senate Committee on Finance. 1970. *Medicare and Medicaid—Problems, Issues, and Alternatives.* 91st Cong., 1st sess. Washington: Government Printing Office.

Senate Special Committee on Aging. 1971. *Developments in Aging, 1970.* 92nd Cong., 1st sess. Washington: Government Printing Office.

Shapiro, S.; Steinwachs, D.M.; Skinner, E.H.; and Mushlin, A.I. 1976. *Survey of Quality Assurance and Utilization Review Mechanisms in Prepaid Group Practice Plans and Medical Care Foundations.* Baltimore: Health Services Research and Development Center, Johns Hopkins Medical Institutions.

Sherwood, S. 1975. Long-term care issues, perspectives, and directions. In *Long-Term Care—A Handbook for Researchers, Planners, and Providers,* S. Sherwood, ed., pp. 3-80. New York: Spectrum/Halsted Press.

Storey, P.B., and Roth, R.B. 1971. Emergency medical care in the Soviet Union: a study of the Skoraya. *JAMA* 217:588-92.

Stotsky, B.A. 1970. *The Nursing Home and the Aged Patient.* New York: Appleton Century Crofts.

Tenney, J.B.; White, K.L.; and Williamson, J.W. 1974. *National Ambulatory Care Survey: Background and Methodology. United States—1967-1972.* National Center for Health Statistics, Vital and Health Statistics, Series 2, No. 61. Rockville, Md.: Department of Health, Education and Welfare, Publication No. (HRA) 74-1335.

Trussell, R.E.; Morehead, M.A.; and Ehrlich, J. 1962. *The Quantity, Quality and Costs of Medical and Hospital Care Secured by a Sample of Teamster Families in the New York Area.* New York: Columbia University School of Public Health and Administrative Medicine.

Weinerman, E.R.; Ratner, R.S.; Robbins, A.; and Lavenhar, M.A. 1966. Yale studies in ambulatory medical care, pt. 5: Determinants of use of hospital emergency services. *Am J Public Health* 56:1037-56.

White, K.L. 1973. Life and death and medicine. *Sci Am* 229(3):23-33.

———. 1974. Health care organization: Trends and opportunities. *Am J Dis Child* 127:549-53.

Wilder, C.S. 1972. *Physician Visits—Volume and Interval Since Last Visit.* National Center for Health Statistics, Vital and Health Statistics, Series 10, No. 75. Rockville, Md.: Department of Health, Education and Welfare, Publication No. (HRA) 72-1064.

Wyler, A.R.; Masuda, M.; and Holmes, T.H. 1971. Magnitude of life events and seriousness of illness. *Psychosom Med* 33:115-22.

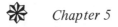 *Chapter 5*

Managing Quality Assurance Information Needs: A Brief Introduction to Structured Group Judgment and Problems of Health Sciences Information

It was proposed in Chapter 1 that the management of information problems in quality assurance is an area of substantial improvement potential. A definitive solution to the problems of health sciences information may not be available or even feasible, given the rapid growth of related fields. However, some strategies for dealing with them are immediately at hand and seem well worth considering. The following will outline several of these strategies, together with some tentative evidence regarding their validity and reliability. Special attention will be given to the use of structured group judgment techniques, particularly as applied to two vital functions:

- The identification, with as much precision as possible, of where in the broad range of health care activities quality assurance effort might have the greatest impact;
- The development of valid and acceptable standards for the measurement of outcomes of care.

At present, the major priorities for local quality assurance activity are often based on the policy decisions of national agencies, such as the Professional Standards Review Organizations or the Joint Commission on Accreditation of Hospitals, although the impact of these decisions on improving patient health and reducing care costs remains open to question (Institute of Medicine, 1976). However, both agencies authorize local providers to establish their own priorities in selecting individual topics and develop standards for required quality assurance projects. While content considerations are important—for example health problem prevalence, seriousness of untreated problems, efficacy of treatment or preventive care, and possibly utilization and fiscal factors (cf. Chapter 4)—a more immediate consideration is the decision process by which such priorities are established. Who should set priorities and standards for measurement, what data are required, and how should judgments be elicited? These critical decisions are often made arbitrarily by one individual or by small groups in informal discussion. Consequently, the information base for such decisions will more often than not be limited, required efficacy and value judgments will be implicit and unchallenged, and the bias of status and authority will be dominant.

THE VALUE OF STRUCTURED GROUP JUDGMENT

It has been long recognized that two heads are better than one. Dalkey suggests that a practical extension of this aphorism might be that *"n* heads are better than one" (Dalkey et al., 1972), based on the assumption that the intelligence of a group can and should be greater than the sum of the individual intelligences making up the group. There is, thus, a potential interaction effect that can lead to a much broader base of facts, ideas, analytic considerations, and innovative syntheses than could be obtained from consulting each member alone. However, it is equally well recognized that committees and forums can be among the most counterproductive of man's institutions. Thousands of manhours may be wasted in semantic arguments and manipulations and in juggling for status, power, or personal recognition. The actual purpose for which many groups are assembled may never be explicitly stated or have much influence on the course of the group interaction.

There is thus much justifiable skepticism regarding the efficiency and effectiveness of traditional, informal small group decision making. Asch (1958) and Dahl (1974) have summarized the usual problems faced by such bodies: a dominant individual may inhibit others; group opinion is influenced to a disproportionate degree by the person who talks most; often the communication in a discussion group has more to do with individual interests than with problem solving; most group members prefer to share only well developed ideas; many find it less threatening to react to the ideas of others than to generate their own; traditional interactive groups often focus on narrow subject areas, sometimes restricting themselves to those ideas put forth earliest in the meeting; topics tend to be obvious and unimportant rather than meaningful and vital; premature evaluation of problems is common; there is difficulty in exploring problem dimensions; and finally, the group itself exerts pressure for conformity as opposed to creativity.

A relatively recent approach involving the use of structured group judgment techniques has been developed to address these problems. Delphi and nominal group methods are illustrations of this trend. Since research or other empirically validated data are lacking for many of the information needs outlined in Chapter 1 and the validity of existing information and hypotheses is frequently in question, this new field may have much to offer to quality assurance and policy staff. Its techniques may prove both efficient and effective for decision making and policy formulation under current conditions of informational uncertainty and in the face of continuous and accelerating social, scientific, and technological change.

The development of formal techniques for eliciting group judgments began in the early 1950s with the work of Dalkey and Helmer. Out of this experience grew the Delphi method of systematic use of expert judgment, a procedure utilizing panels that never meet face to face (Dalkey et al., 1972; Dalkey, 1969). A comprehensive description of the technique, especially as adapted to policy purposes, has been given by Linstone and Turoff (1975). Small group judgment techniques were formalized in the late 1960s (Delbecq and Van de Ven, 1967, 1971; Van de Ven and Delbecq, 1971, 1972). These nominal group techniques usually require small groups and encompass formal procedures to reduce the bias that is inherent in open, interactive, and nonstructured group processes (Delbecq, Van de Ven, and Gustafson, 1975). Also, several investigators (Dahl, 1974; Gustafson et al., 1973; Dalkey et al., 1972) have been able to demonstrate that more valid information can be extracted from a group by using formal techniques and that a greater quantity of useful data can be generated. The evidence on this point could have important implications for organizational problem solving and development.

FORMAL GROUP JUDGMENT TECHNIQUES IN QUALITY ASSURANCE

In the following, the use of systematic group judgment is recommended for purposes of establishing both cost-effective assessment topics and outcome standards for identifying deficient care. Group judgments regarding health problem prevalence, treatment efficacy, and current level of performance are essential for such purposes. To optimize the results of formal group judgment in quality assurance, four basic functions of this technique must be recognized:

- Establishing team composition,
- Determining team size,
- Specifying required information, and
- Eliciting team judgments.

Team Composition

Establishing team composition in terms of the background of its members is the first major function. The relevance and validity of the knowledge and experiential base represented by the group may well determine the quality of their collective judgment. Quality assurance activity requires knowledge and experience in three general areas that are the basis of nearly all health care decisions and therefore must be adequately reflected by a quality assurance group: (1) relevant medical science information; (2) local care content and performance (patients, problems, resources, and clinical management); and (3) the value systems of local consumers and providers. This base is essential for establishing priorities for assessment and improvement, for developing standards and valid measures of care outcomes and processes, and for developing effective improvement strategies if deficiencies are identified.

The first consideration in team composition is based on the fact that adequate and relevant medical science information, knowledge of the efficacy and safety of therapeutic interventions, and awareness of the limits of validity of diagnostic methods are crucial prerequisites to quality assurance planning. This requires the inclusion of team members with medical expertise and considerable knowledge of health care research relevant to the concerns of the provider institution. Awareness of information that is applicable to local care problems, as well as the ability to judge the scientific credibility and validity of published information, is required. While most local health care institutions will not usually have recognized experts at their disposal, they will generally count among their staff some members who have taken a special interest in certain aspects of the field and can serve as a scientific monitor in group deliberations. Another possibility is to invite an outside specialist to sit on the quality assurance team. This can be an exceptional means of meeting the scientific information needs of the group and may prove to be of far greater impact for the institution overall than having the same expert give a staff lecture in traditional continuing education programs.

The second consideration, local care content and performance, requires local experience in terms of patients, health problems, provider and community resources, and probable levels of current performance. This calls for team members with overall familiarity with the provider institution. Identifying topics for quality assurance activity requires that the team consist of at least four physicians, primarily generalists, to provide a core group with knowledge of aspects of efficacy and prognosis. Nurses, technicians, or even front desk personnel should also be included; an administrator familiar with the fiscal aspects of care is an especially valuable team member, as most quality assurance requires a series of cost-effectiveness decisions. Special emphasis must be given to obtaining valid judgments regarding present care deficiencies in areas where there is adequate evidence of health care efficacy. In view of the constraints on most quality assurance resources, it is a serious but avoidable error to spend substantial effort on evaluating outcomes or processes of care only to find that standards are being met or that nothing can be done to improve performance for lack of interventions or procedures of established efficacy. The identification of serious correctable deficiencies of care provides a validation of initial group judgments in selecting a given topic. Consequently, a vital consideration in choosing team members is to obtain the most valid experiential estimates regarding the probable quality of current performance.

The third consideration in selecting a quality assurance team is to provide a range of experience that reflects the value systems of both consumers and providers. Usually, most providers will adequately represent local institutional as well as individual staff values. What is usually neglected are members who represent consumer, if not overall societal, values. Such value considerations, however, relate directly to the identification of priorities for assessment topics, as well as to the setting of standards of accomplishment that are reasonable within the limits of local resources. The statement of such values can also have economic and social advantages, as it permits consideration of the effects of consumer relations and patient satisfaction on quality of care. Again, the inclusion of nonphysician members on the provider staff is the very least that can be done to meet this requirement. A sophisticated lay person offers the additional advantage of providing an effective challenge to provider assumptions, and seemingly naive questions often provoke rethinking of cherished but untested professional premises and prejudices.

Determination of Team Size

The size of the group to be organized for quality assurance or, for that matter, for any decision making depends primarily upon whether or not the group will meet face to face. Group judgment processes as here recommended require a series of meetings during which responses are elicited, aggregated, and resubmitted to the group for a subsequent round of judgment and response (Williamson, 1978).

If team members do not meet together, the use of large numbers can be an advantage in eliciting a wide spectrum of ideas. Direct mail questionnaires are usual for such large groups, but personal interviews could conceivably fill the same purpose. More practical methods such as "computer conferencing" are being developed and may facilitate large group interactions (Turoff, 1976). Dalkey has studied the relation of group size to the reliability and validity of team estimates of obscure data, such as the number of telephones in use in Africa in 1965, and has demonstrated a direct correlation between group size and the reliability as well as accuracy of team estimates (Dalkey et al., 1972).

For quality assurance conducted within institutions, face-to-face meetings or sequential interviews have proven a practical means of applying structured decision methods. There is substantial evidence that five to thirteen members probably constitute the lower and upper limits of group size (Emlet et al., 1971a; Dalkey, 1969; Delbecq, 1968; Bales and Borgatta, 1955). Having less than five members restricts the experiential base of the group; having more than thirteen results in such complex group dynamics that time factors alone tend to preclude adequate participation from each member.

Specification of Required Information
The validity of group judgments under conditions of informational uncertainty can be enhanced by any factual input, however limited (Dalkey, Brown, and Cochrane, 1970). In the above example of group estimation of obscure data, such as the number of telephones in Africa, information regarding the population of Africa or the number of telephones in Algeria seems to have notably improved the validity of the estimates (Dalkey et al., 1972). Clearly, use of structured group judgment methods for quality assurance will be facilitated by the provision of as much accurate and relevant data and literature as possible; for example, information regarding numbers of patients seen in the facility or other provider setting; their diagnoses and demographic characteristics; listings of provider characteristics in terms of physicians, physician extenders, nurses, and technicians; utilization statistics; results of any previous quality assurance or assessment studies in the institution; and any particularly relevant literature. It is the author's experience that a surprising amount of valuable information is buried in clinic or hospital archives that

might be meaningful in terms of quality assurance, such as administrative records or committee reports on problems related to the
assessment of care.

The information required for group judgment in quality assurance
can be roughly divided according to the following five assessment
and improvement stages. Although specifically relating to the
methods of health accounting (see Chapters 6–10), these stages reflect
basic quality assurance categories and apply as well to the medical
care evaluation studies of the Professional Standards Review Organizations and the performance evaluation procedures of the Joint
Commission on Accreditation of Hospitals.

The selection of quality assurance priorities requires consideration
of the spectrum of topics that might be studied with a view to improvement of effectiveness of care (especially in terms of patient
health outcomes) or of its efficiency (especially in terms of resource
utilization). The main purpose at this stage is to identify assessment
topics having the greatest achievable benefit not being achieved in
present practice (see Chapter 3 for a discussion of this concept).
Finding acceptable evidence in the health sciences literature of the
improvement of outcomes will stimulate inquiry into whether similar
problems, similarly amenable to such solutions, exist locally. On the
other hand, literature confirming the existence of deficiencies for
which significant improvement has not yet been documented may
alert the team to the practical limits of quality assessment. If the
staff of any institution can be alerted to methods of searching the
literature for meaningful topics of local quality assurance activity,
much valuable material may become available to the priority setting
team.

Initial outcome assessment involves the selection of outcomes that
may offer the greatest improvement potential in regard to the priority topic chosen and the design of practical means for assessing them.
Here, the information need is for outcome assessment methods and
their advantages and disadvantages. Greene (1976) has provided one
of the more authoritative discussions of assessment methods and related considerations; a recent review by the Institute of Medicine of
the National Academy of Sciences (1976) presents a thorough analysis of current methods and systems of health care assessment; and
The Johns Hopkins Center for Health Services Research (Shapiro et
al., 1976) has reviewed and analyzed quality assessment methods
related to group practice in ambulatory care. This and similar literature can provide helpful insights into the problems of organizing
assessment studies, developing standards and measures, and interpreting the results.

Definitive assessment requires the verification of deficiencies singled out by initial assessment and identification of specific correctable determinants. Here the information base is more complex. Few quality assessment methods claim to identify inadequate performance or outcomes. They nearly always stipulate that if measured care does not meet accepted standards, subsequent analysis is necessary to confirm whether a true deficiency exists. This is important, as problems may not be due to staff performance but rather to unalterable circumstances or even to errors of assessment. However, an increasing number of authors, e.g., Rutstein et al. (1976), have discussed and documented preventable case fatalities or disabilities that might be directly related to inadequate performance, and some have provided useful outcome standards for specific deficiencies (Avery et al., 1976). Critical incident studies are especially good sources of such information. Sanazaro and Williamson (1970) have provided a systematic outline of reported preventable errors and achieved successes in contemporary medical care throughout the United States.

Improvement involves the planning and implementation of concrete measures to correct established deficiencies. The literature in this respect is rather sparse and difficult to retrieve (Williamson, 1977). The problems of effecting meaningful behavioral or organizational change are complex and difficult to evaluate. Too often, when care deficiencies are identified and confirmed, the quality assurance group recommends an informational approach, on the assumption that all that is necessary is to tell the staff to "go and sin no more." Continuing medical education by exhortation has rarely been found effective in achieving substantial and sustained improvement, however. Clearly, it is essential that quality assurance teams obtain at least some evidence of the probable effectiveness of proposed improvement actions and of the advantages of one improvement modality over others for the specific problem to be solved.

The evaluation of impact requires reassessment to see if standards are now being met and verification of the effectiveness of the measures taken in producing observed improvements. If institutional or organizational changes have been made, the problem of attribution to quality assurance activity may be explicit and unquestioned. However, most education efforts and administrative changes probably do not permit such straightforward interpretation. Impact evaluation designs are often inadequate or do not permit of generalization beyond the cases studied. Usually, the main problem is one of obtaining valid evidence for the attribution of observed change to the improvement measures implemented. In a review of literature on continuing medical education evaluation, Bertram and Brooks-

Bertram (1977) found that of 113 reported evaluation studies, 8 were scientifically supportable, and of these, only 3 confirmed improvement lasting at least six weeks. A review of consumer health education literature is equally pessimistic (Werlin, 1976). Again, the major failing is lack of adequate evidence permitting the attribution of measured improvements to the actions taken.

The information requirements of each quality assurance project will have to be considered individually and with a view to these stages, and the probable cost balanced against the potential benefits of effort expended on obtaining information. Whatever the effort, it will enhance the ultimate impact of quality assurance activity.

Eliciting Team Judgments

A number of different methods can be applied to structuring the procedures for eliciting group judgments. In a collaborative Health Benefit Analysis study, a large number of options were developed, each having different advantages and disadvantages depending upon the goals to be accomplished (Emlet et al., 1971a, 1971b). Two major categories of methods for eliciting team judgments have received considerable attention. In contrast to the Delphi method (Linstone and Turoff, 1975; Dalkey, 1969) described previously, the nominal group technique (Delbecq, Van de Ven, and Gustafson, 1975) involves small groups who meet face to face. Structured procedures for eliciting group judgment are used, the procedures varying according to the information needed. The estimation of data can rely on a somewhat different approach from that used in developing policy options, as it does not require methods for the clarification of values. All of these methods, however, are based on the assumption that, among any similarly qualified group, it is impossible to identify one member whose responses would represent the most valid or meaningful judgment. Therefore, the best strategy is to rely on the aggregate judgment of the group as a whole.

For quality assurance purposes, a modified nominal group process for eliciting team judgment is recommended to achieve the most effective results with the least expenditure of effort. The demonstrated advantages of a structured topic selection process as applied in a series of quality assurance projects conducted by health accounting methods (Williamson, 1978) can be summarized as follows:

- Structured methods for eliciting group judgment provide improved benefits of care for both providers and patients by stimulating internally motivated staff involvement in more creative and meaningful quality assurance activity.

- These methods seem to be successful in broadening the perspective of participating personnel to a more holistic and cost-effective view of problems.
- When health is the target benefit, this process has led to greater emphasis on overall prevention, health maintenance, and patient management as opposed to emphasis on curative management of specific organic disease.
- Topics selected by these methods direct the attention of the quality assurance teams to a variety of innovative and challenging methods for assessing and improving health care.
- The priority judgment process is more effective because it forces consideration of salient local care factors specific to a facility; of local patient or administrative data as well as national information; and of staff assumptions regarding efficacy of care interventions and the likelihood of achieving behavioral or organizational change.

The disadvantages of the proposed method should also be considered:

- Formal group processes are often unfamiliar to staff and, if not handled well, can seem contrived.
- Since a team effort is required, more staff time is involved than would be the case if one person arbitrarily selected all topics.
- The technique works best if the team leader or coordinator is experienced or has been trained by someone familiar with nominal group processes. Locating personnel with such experience is difficult at present, although training manuals are now available (Delbecq, Van de Ven, and Gustafson, 1975).
- The method requires a strong leader who will insist on structured procedures and avoid the natural tendency to revert to the more inefficient though comfortable informal discussion.
- The method can prove emotionally draining, if not anxiety producing, especially if a team member's judgment is consistently outside the range of the judgment of the remaining team members or if cherished assumptions of team members are threatened.

In summary, effective use of structured group judgment in circumstances where adequate research data are lacking can provide the basis for setting valid quality assurance priorities and standards. Practical if limited experience with group judgment approaches was gained in some of the health accounting projects described in Chapters 6-10, which will provide an illustration of preliminary efforts and results in this respect.

PROBLEMS OF HEALTH SCIENCES INFORMATION: RELEVANCE, VALIDITY, AND ACCESSIBILITY

One of the most difficult problems facing a quality assurance team is how to assess the relevance, validity, and accessibility of the health sciences information that is required at each quality assurance stage. The sheer volume of published material is overwhelming, and the number of new journal titles alone is increasing rapidly. For the purposes of quality assurance, moreover, much of this information is probably irrelevant, invalid, or inaccessible physically or conceptually. How then can a quality assurance team deal with these problems?

Judging the relevance of available information requires developing some familiarity with the overall field of quality assurance, its key concepts, and the specific functions of assessment and improvement of care. Quality assurance teams planning prospective outcome assessment will find relevant information in publications on sampling and survey methods, questionnaire design, and response and completion rates. The development of outcome standards, especially those encompassing health outcomes, will both require and foster an understanding of the natural history of disease processes, including the course of patient functional disabilities and treated prognoses, and of the harmfulness or inutility of some current health care practices. This in turn should lead to an understanding of important measurable outcomes. On the other hand, the quality assurance team will soon discover that the multitude of isolated, unreplicated clinical reports and case studies that pervade the current literature may have very little immediate applicability in clinical practice, let alone being of use for developing either process or outcome standards. Even worse are the numerous conflicting reports based on studies of discrepant patient populations, lacking uniform descriptions of the health problem and any description of the providers, which make generalization to other populations difficult if not meaningless.

The main point, however, is that much valuable information relevant to quality assurance is available if sought and found. Recognizing the general literature field to search, knowing what headings to look up, and understanding the jargon encompassed in such reports is a difficult but not impossible task (Williamson, 1977).

Addressing the problem of whether relevant health sciences information is also valid for the intended quality assurance purpose can be a highly technical task. Interpreting the adequacy of statistical analyses or analyzing the research design or the adequacy of data collection requires a fair amount of research sophistication. Moreover, many reports include inadequate documentation in these respects. The most reliable information for the quality assurance team will generally come from analyses by independent expert panels, for example, the drug efficacy panels of the National Research Council and of the Food and Drug Administration. Publications such as the *Medical Letter* are sources of valuable information in coping with the problem of data validity and proof of efficacy in relation to drugs and pharmaceuticals. Several surveys have indicated that the average practitioner utilizes drug company detail men as a primary source of drug information, a practice that raises serious questions of information bias. These issues are discussed by Burack and Fox (1976), whose exposition is well documented and sufficiently factual to allow quality assurance staff to formulate their own conclusions from the data presented. Other authors (e.g., Colton, 1974) have addressed the statistical problems of interpreting published literature and have provided practical guidelines for this purpose.

While a detailed examination of the validity, or lack of it, of current biomedical and health sciences literature is beyond the scope and purpose of this discussion, the following items are suggested as a relatively simple if crude tool for assessing the validity of reported research findings (Williamson, 1977):

- Is the author reporting work in the field of his own expertise and experience?
- What evaluative comments are available from colleagues, experts, or published reviews?
- What is the reputation and editorial policy of the publisher of the article?
- What is the source of the data or information upon which the report is based?
  Primary rather than secondary sources should be obtained wherever possible.
  Primary research reports can be more validly judged than summaries, although reports by expert panels are an exception to this.
- Has the research been replicated?
  If replicated, what is the extent of agreement among independent investigators?
- If an experimental study is described,
  Was health problem content specified in terms of criteria for inclusion and exclusion of experimental subjects?
  Was a control group used in the design?

Was there random allocation of the experimental treatment between control and experimental subjects?
Were the experimental and control groups studied concurrently?
Was a double blind design used in evaluating the results?
Was the response rate adequate to justify generalization?
- If diagnostic validation studies are described,
How valid is the criterion against which the experimental procedure is to be tested?
Are both false negative (e.g., missed diagnosis) and false positive (e.g., misdiagnosis) rates computed and stated?
Was the method for computing the false negative and false positive rates indicated?
Was the standard indicating acceptable limits of the rate of false negatives and false positives stated?
- If an epidemiological study is described,
Is the specific population sampled adequately described?
Is the method of sampling described in some detail?
Were substitution methods used to replace those in the original sample who could not be contacted?
Was the response rate high enough to support generalization?
If a survey was based on a questionnaire, was it pretested for communication effectiveness and were reliability–validity test coefficients determined?
- Is there adequate information to evaluate the statistical analysis utilized?
Was the statistical test used named or described?
Were assumptions related to the test mentioned in the study?
Was the level of statistical significance made explicit?

Finally, there is the problem of gaining access to needed information, which is often one of logistics and labeling. Much relevant and valid information is available but is frequently conceptually inaccessible; in other words, needed information and data are there, whether in libraries or computer archives, but are classified under headings or described in terms that are difficult to recognize except for those specialized in a given field.

Heading the list of essential quality assurance literature is that providing evidence of causal relations between medical care outcomes and processes and describing the limits of validity of diagnostic interventions and the efficacy and safety of therapeutic interventions. Relevant and valid literature may become more accessible for quality assurance if some key labeling concepts suggested in the following list can be recognized (Williamson, 1977):

Critical incident studies
Process determinants of outcomes
Health care benefits (or disbenefits)
Unnecessary or neglected health care
Clinical observer error
Utilization determinants
Cost-benefit studies
Quality assessment standards, criteria, and norms
Validated quality assessment standards
Algorithms, protocols, and decision trees
Diagnostic reliability or validity
Therapeutic reliability and validity
Controlled clinical trials
Natural history studies
Longitudinal studies
Treated prognosis (or clinical prognosis)

It is obvious that most of these terms will not be found in any one index or indexing system. Many come from widely different fields of scholarship; for example, critical incident studies are most often found in the education literature, cost-benefit studies in the economic literature, controlled clinical trials in the biomedical research literature, and quality assessment methods in the health services research literature.

Another common information need for which much data exist relates to the prevalence of health problems managed in the ambulatory or institutional practice of U.S. physicians. *The Vital and Health Statistics* compilations of the various national health surveys of the National Center for Health Statistics provide some of the best data available in this area. The National Ambulatory Medical Care Survey, for example, provides yearly cross-sectional data for several factors related to private office practice in this country, of which the tabulations of patient complaints, symptoms, and problems that bring them to the physician are of obvious relevance to quality assurance. Equally valuable are the tabulations of physician diagnoses of the major problems identified, rated as to seriousness of likely impairment if untreated, the number of minutes of physician care rendered, whether laboratory tests were ordered or treatment prescribed, and final disposition. Surveys of hospital discharges provide equally valuable statistics on diagnoses, length of stay, and diagnostic and therapeutic management provided. The major drawback of such national health statistics for local quality assurance teams is that they relate to the entire United States population. However, the use of small group judgment methods might provide a reasonable place to start if extrapolations to local population groups are to be made.

Finally, data regarding care costs are vital to cost-effectiveness assessment. Surprisingly little is usually available from local administrative records, due to the absence of unit costing by specific health problems (Sorensen, 1976) or by patient or provider groups related to topics relevant to quality assurance. Institutional totals that are available often have little application to specific studies. Some valuable national data are provided by the Office of Research and Statistics of the Social Security Administration, although these have the same limitations as other national health statistics regarding their applicability to local populations. Again, careful extrapolation can provide a valuable data base for local quality assurance teams.

SUMMARY

The success of quality assurance will in large degree depend on an effective management of health information needs which will allow the selection of topics encompassing achievable health benefit not achieved in current practice. It follows that analysis of this selection process will provide crucial information for determining the eventual cost effectiveness and impact of quality assurance projects. In this chapter, nominal group processes for eliciting consensual team judgments have been advocated as providing an efficient framework for this approach, based on evidence of the advantages of such methods over nonstructured open group interactions.

Several procedural considerations have been outlined, including the selection of the most qualified priority and standard setting teams, composed of a core of physicians but including other health professionals and lay persons; the use of formal procedures for eliciting judgments required in priority and standard setting, in assessing and improving performance, and in evaluating results; and finally, the use of a selective approach to health sciences literature to cope with the problem of the relevance, validity, and accessibility of required information.

The findings and conclusions of a number of health accounting projects, reported in Part II of this book and elsewhere (Williamson, 1978; Williamson et al., 1978), have provided evidence of the feasibility of planning and conducting assessment studies on a wide variety of topics that are not limited to existing health information systems but use prospective followup surveys of patients to establish health outcomes. It is the author's belief, based on this experience, that the goals of quality assurance will probably not be realized until assessment of important problems goes beyond the narrow confines of available data and current health information.

REFERENCES

Asch, S.C. 1958. Effects of group pressure upon the modification and distortion of judgments. In *Readings in Social Psychology*, 3rd ed., E. Macoby, T. Newcomb and E. Hartley, eds., pp. 174-83. New York: Holt, Rinehardt and Winston.

Avery, A.D.; Lelah, T.; Solomon, N.E.; Harris, L.J.; Brook, R.H.; Greenfield, S.; Ware, J.E.; and Avery, C.H. 1976. *Quality of Medical Care Assessment Using Outcome Measures: Eight Disease-Specific Applications.* R-2021/2HEW. Santa Monica, Cal.: Rand.

Bales, R.F., and Borgatta, E.F. 1955. Size of group as a factor in the interaction profile. In *Small Groups: Studies in Social Interaction*, A.P. Hare, E.F. Borgatta, and R.F. Bales, eds., pp. 396-413. New York: Knopf.

Bertram, D., and Brooks-Bertram, P. 1977. *The Evaluation of Continuing Medical Education—A Literature Review.* Health Education Monographs, vol. 5, no. 4. Baltimore: Department of Health Education, The Johns Hopkins School of Hygiene and Public Health.

Burack, R., and Fox, F.J. 1976. *The 1976 Handbook of Prescription Drugs.* New York: Random House.

Colton, T. 1974. *Statistics in Medicine.* Boston: Little, Brown.

Dahl, A.W. 1974. Delphi and interactive committee processes in a comprehensive health planning advisory council: a comparative case study. Doctoral thesis, The Johns Hopkins University School of Hygiene and Public Health.

Dalkey, N.C. 1969. *The Delphi Method—An Experimental Study of Group Opinion.* Memorandum RM-5888-PR. Santa Monica, Cal.: Rand.

Dalkey, N.C.; Brown, B.; and Cochrane, S. 1970. *The Delphi Method.* Pt. 4: *Effect of Percentile Feedback and Feed-In of Relevant Facts.* Memorandum RM-6118-PR. Santa Monica, Cal.: Rand

Dalkey, N.C., ed.; Rourke, D.L.; Lewis, R.; and Snyder, S. 1972. *Studies in the Quality of Life—Delphi and Decision-Making.* Lexington, Mass: Lexington Books/Heath.

Delbecq, A.L. 1968. The world within the "span of control"—Managerial behavior in groups of varied size. *Business Horizons* 10(4):47-56.

Delbecq, A.L., and Van de Ven, A.H. 1967. Nominal group techniques for involving clients and resource experts in program planning. Academy of Management Proceedings. Seattle: Graduate School of Business Administration, University of Washington.

———. 1971. A group process model for problem identification and program planning. *J Appl Behav Sci* 7:466-92.

Delbecq, A.L.; Van de Ven, A.H.; and Gustafson, D.H. 1975. *Group Techniques for Program Planning.* Glenview, Ill.: Scott, Foresman.

Emlet, H.E.; Williamson, J.W.; Casey, I.; and Davis, J. L. 1971a. *Alternative*

Methods for Estimating Health Care Benefits and Required Resources. Vol. 1: *Summary.* Falls Church, Va.: Analytic Services.

Emlet, H.E.; Davis, J.L.; and Casey, I. 1971b. *Alternative Methods for Estimating Health Care Benefits and Required Resources.* Vol. 2: *Selecting the Estimators.* Falls Church, Va.: Analytic Services.

Greene, R. 1976. *Assuring Quality in Medical Care—State of the Art.* Cambridge, Mass.: Ballinger.

Gustafson, D.H.; Shukla, R.K.; Delbecq, A.L.; and Walster, G.W. 1973. A comparative study of differences in subjective likelihood estimates made by individuals, interacting groups, Delphi groups and nominal groups. *Organizational Behavior and Human Performance* 9:280–91.

Institute of Medicine. 1976. *Assessing Quality in Health Care—An Evaluation.* Washington: National Academy of Sciences.

Linstone, H.A., and Turoff, M., eds. 1975. *The Delphi Method—Techniques and Applications.* Reading, Mass.: Addison-Wesley.

Rutstein, D.D.; Berenberg, W.; Chalmers, T.C.; Child, C.G.; Fishman, A.P.; and Perrin, E.B. 1976. Measuring the quality of medical care—a clinical method. *N Engl J Med* 294:582–88.

Sanazaro, P.J., and Williamson, J.W. 1970. Physician performance and its effects on patients—a classification based on reports by internists, surgeons, pediatricians and obstetricians. *Med Care* 8:299–308.

Shapiro, S.; Steinwachs, D.M.; Skinner, E.H.; and Mushlin, A.I. 1976. *Survey of Quality Assurance and Utilization Review Mechanisms in Prepaid Group Practice Plans and Medical Care Foundations.* Baltimore: Health Services Research and Development Center, Johns Hopkins Medical Institutions.

Sorensen, J.E. 1976. Uniform cost accounting in long-term care. In *Long-Term Care Data, Report on the Conference on Long-Term Health Care Data,* J. Murnaghan, ed., pp. 154–59. Philadelphia: Lippincott. Reprinted from *Med Care* 14(5) Supplement.

Turoff, M. 1976. The design of a policy Delphi. *Technological Forecasting and Social Change* 2:149–71.

Van de Ven, A.H., and Delbecq, A.L. 1971. Nominal and interacting group processes for committee decision-making effectiveness. *Acad Man J* 14:203–12.

———. 1972. The nominal group as a research instrument for exploratory health studies. *Am J Public Health* 62:337–42.

Werlin, S.H. 1976. *A Survey of Consumer Health Education Programs.* Cambridge, Mass.: Arthur B. Little.

Williamson, J.W. 1977. *Improving Medical Practice and Health Care—A Bibliographic Guide to Information Management in Quality Assurance.* Cambridge, Mass.: Ballinger.

———. 1978. Formulating priorities for quality assurance activity—description of a method and its application. *JAMA:* 239:631–37.

Williamson, J.W.; Braswell, H.R.; Horn, S.D.; and Lohmeyer, S. 1978. Priority setting in quality assurance: Reliability of staff judgment in medical institutions. *Med Care* (in press).

✳ *Part II*

Health Accounting—Description and Results of an Outcome Based Quality Assurance Strategy

Chapter 6

The Origin and Structure of Health Accounting

The health accounting approach to quality assurance is based on the assumption that any single method or restriction to a specific data base will be of limited usefulness because of the wide range of local institutional characteristics and needs and of the continuing evolution of methods for assessing and improving health services. Therefore, among its basic aims was and is the education of health care providers in some of the essential principles and strategies for assessment and improvement of performance and in the resources and skills necessary for an active involvement in quality assurance functions.

ORGANIZATION AND DEVELOPMENT

In the following, the origins, the organizational development, and the methods of health accounting as an outcome based strategy for quality assurance will be presented for three separate periods: 1963–1966, 1966–1969, and 1969–1973. Each period represents an independent phase, with different specific goals and sources of funding, although the overall purpose remained the development of a conceptual and procedural basis for constructing ongoing systems of health care outcome assessment and improvement. Some of the study priorities and procedures of the early participants in this endeavor may seem inappropriate in the light of our more recent experiences, but many of their findings still seem remarkably relevant, and the institutional and organizational aspects of the early health accounting projects may provide many valuable insights. In particular, with regard to such basic problems as physician and institutional motivation and interest in quality of care aspects, the organizational successes and failures of that phase may well be as instructive as the assessment and improvement methods and results that have evolved.

The Origins of Health Accounting—
1963-1966

From 1963 to 1966, the initial framework of health accounting was developed, and a series of outcome studies were developed and implemented. A remarkable group of university students became involved during this period who would later play a major role in shaping quality assurance in the United States. Also during these years, the conceptual framework of health accounting was accepted by the American Medical Association as the basis for reorganizing their National Plan for Continuing Medical Education (Storey, Williamson, and Castle, 1968).

Integrating Assessment of Patient Care with Continuing Medical Education. The initial concepts of health accounting were based on research into the systematic evaluation and improvement of health care outcomes related to specific population groups. At the time, integrating research in patient care and continuing education of health care practitioners seemed a meaningful direction, as reflected in these four basic assumptions (Williamson, 1962):

- To be effective, the continuing medical education curriculum must be based on knowledge of the specific educational needs of physicians.
- A physician's subjective evaluation of his educational needs is probably an inadequate approximation of his real needs.
- Learning motivation is probably best obtained by making the physician aware of his specific educational needs through impersonal and objective methods of measurement that could be periodically applied throughout the span of his career.
- There are few if any objective means of evaluating competence of medical performance and delineating specific educational needs, and indeed, this is probably the single most important area of research and development in continuing medical education.

The development and implementation of the first phase of health accounting took place at the University of Illinois School of Medicine in Chicago, in collaboration with the Rockford Community

Hospital and an associated multispecialty group clinic located in Rockford, Illinois, a city of about 150,000 people. In 1963, the hospital staff sought assistance from the university in developing new policy directions for their continuing medical education programs. The hospital staff were questioning the effectiveness of their continuing education policy, and a request to the state School of Medicine led to a formal agreement between the hospital and the medical school under which the hospital collaborated in methodological studies of the assessment of medical practice, with the object of identifying specific educational objectives for achieving patient health improvement.

Advisory groups were organized in both the community hospital and the university, and this administrative arrangement provided the setting for the first nine health accounting projects. Building on the Rockford experience, an additional project (Gonnella et al., 1970), in which members of the School of Medicine of the University of Illinois cooperated, demonstrated an outcome approach for assessing medical care in an outpatient clinic.

What is important to note is the fact that the community hospital staff came to the university on their own. On its side, the university, being a land grant college, was under statutory obligation to participate in offering continuing medical education to the community to which it was responsible. Both groups were thus motivated to collaborate, and the point of departure was their willingness to break away from the traditional approach—i.e., by communicating through journal articles and formal continuing education courses—to the problem of improving health care. Their willingness to experiment educationally was due in large measure to the available resources and innovative atmosphere created by the staff of the Office of Research in Medical Education, supported by a program grant from the Commonwealth Fund of New York. This proved to be an effective combination, constituting what may well have been one of the earliest formal research programs in this country in quality assurance as presently defined; that is, research focusing on the integration of health care assessment and improvement functions. Most prior research had concentrated either on assessment of health care or on separate continuing medical education and administrative programs to effect improvement of medical practice.

At the same time, there was concern that proposed programs for continuing medical education (Dryer, 1962), while offering a mass education resource, were almost totally lacking in objective means for identifying educational needs in terms of health care performance deficiency, let alone population health deficiencies. The evolving concepts and methods of health accounting seemed to provide an operational framework for meeting some of these needs, and a program was implemented under the sponsorship of the American Medical Association that involved an initial survey of physician practice, including an epidemiological profile of patients and the problems they presented. Immediate interests and activities in continuing education on the part of the physician were also surveyed. Based on this information, assessment tools were to be developed permitting the objective determination of correctable care deficiencies that seemed most closely related to health outcomes. Experience in this program with a number of national panels organized to develop assessment instruments and judgment-based criteria for relating care processes to health outcomes proved a valuable starting point (Storey, Williamson, and Castle, 1968).

Focus on the Potential for Improvement of Health Care Outcomes. Three basic requirements or organizing principles for an effective quality assurance strategy evolved during the first period of health accounting:

- Integration of systematic health care assessment and improvement stages in a cyclic relationship providing for feedback between stages;
- Initial assessment focus on health care outcomes, with subsequent analysis of related processes only if outcome deficiencies were identified;
- Use of structured small group processes to estimate essential but unavailable data regarding health problem prevalence, efficacy of interventions, and current levels of performance as a basis for establishing assessment topic priorities and outcome standards.

The first of these requirements was tested by actively involving the medical staff at the participating facilities in an inquiry cycle comprising the major elements shown in Figure 6.1; i.e., health care outcome assessment to identify correctable deficiencies and to then estimate the probable impact of improvement action; formulation of objectives for improvement based on evaluation results; and improvement action such as continuing education to overcome deficiencies identified by evaluation and encompassed in the objectives.

In these initial studies, the project leaders at participating health care facilities tended to select study topics related more to the immediate clinical interests of their staff than to more specific health

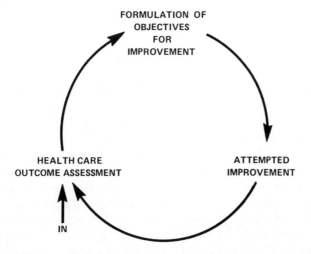

Figure 6.1. The integration of health care outcome assessment and improvement in quality assurance.

outcome topics. The first three projects thus focused on an assessment of the quality of physician responses to abnormal laboratory screening test results, a topic that was both relevant and practicable for one of the principal investigators at the original assessment site, who was chief of pathology at the community hospital where the projects were conducted.

The second organizing principle, relating to the application of an outcome oriented evaluation strategy, required that a specific outcome be measured at one point in time and compared to a standard; if the outcome proved deficient, then associated medical and nonmedical factors were to be systematically examined to single out correctable determinants of the deficient outcome unless and until the study team established that the potential gain was not likely to be worth additional evaluation resources. The initial studies of laboratory data (Williamson, Alexander, and Miller, 1967) proved successful both as an evaluation effort illustrating the outcome assessment approach and as an educational function in terms of achieving staff involvement and willingness to participate in an expanded effort.

In order to develop an adequate information base for establishing quality assurance priorities, three major estimates were considered necessary: the first approximating patient health needs in terms of expected impairment per person times the number of persons in the specific population; the second approximating the extent to which expected health impairment was preventable or remediable; and the third approximating the extent to which impairment considered to be preventable or remediable was in fact being prevented or remedied. However, efforts to obtain measured findings upon which to base these approximations soon revealed an extreme scarcity of data. Health problems had to be categorized by organic disease classification models that were inadequate for assessment purposes even in a hospital setting. The main deficiency was the absence of specific longitudinal data related to patient disabilities and impairment of overall life function. Consequently, it was almost impossible to determine the extent to which the quality of life of individuals or populations had been reduced due to specific health problems.

Available information relating to the efficacy of interventions, whether for curing or caring, proved to be equally inadequate. It soon became clear that such data either did not exist or were so fragmented that even a massive effort would not suffice to retrieve them in usable form. Such information as was found frequently covered only mortality rates, was from unreplicated studies, or provided a contradictory and inadequate basis for establishing reliable assessment priorities and standards. Therefore, a totally different approach appeared to be required. Here, the use of structured small group judgment processes to establish quality assurance topic priorities and outcome assessment standards seemed to offer considerable potential. These procedures, although they were not uniformly applied at least in the initial stages of health accounting, later proved indispensable in data extrapolations to specify study populations and in making explicit team assumptions regarding unavailable information such as health problem prevalence and care efficacy and effectiveness (see Chapter 5 for a discussion of this approach). Briefly, the following steps were involved:

- Selection of a panel incorporating personnel expert in research and patient care for a given health problem;
- Eliciting their judgment regarding the most valid information on problem prevalence, natural history and treated prognoses of health problems, and efficacy of diagnostic and therapeutic interventions; and
- Analysis of the information so elicited for purposes of establishing quality assurance topic priorities and, subsequently, assessment standards.

Research data were to be given the highest priority; next, extrapolated information from indirectly related sources was to be sought; finally, for the vast majority of data needs, factual assumptions were to be made explicit and analyzed, using consensual group judgment methods. This approach, first introduced under the term "prognostic epidemiology" (Williamson, Alexander, and Miller, 1968), yielded the basic methods that were applied in later periods of the health accounting program (Emlet et al., 1973); reformulated as "health benefit analysis" (Williamson and van Nieuwenhuijzen, 1974), they focused on estimating both health benefits and costs of care for specified populations.

Operational Concepts and Approaches— 1966-1969

The second period in the development of health accounting took place at The Johns Hopkins University. Several collaborative studies that were conducted during this period yielded important results. A six level health scale was developed as a standard measurement tool for assessing the overall health and functional status of small population groups. At the same time, the approach to eliciting small group judgments was developed further and extended to the development of outcome standards.

Outcome Assessment by Measures of Overall Health and Functional Status. To permit assessment of patient health outcomes, a standard scale for measuring overall health and functional status across groups of patients was required that would have to meet the following criteria:

- *Independence of health problem type*—The scale should be applicable to all patients regardless of the particular class of their problem.
- *Adaptability to patient age*—In general, the scale should be applicable to patients of any age, ranging from pediatric to geriatric populations.
- *Independence of prognostic considerations*—The scale should measure patient health at any given time regardless of what might happen subsequently.
- *Economy of use*—The scale should permit application with a minimum of financial and personnel resources in a variety of care settings.

The ordinal scale eventually developed on the basis of the impairment and functional disability categories discussed in Chapter 3 included the following six levels:

1. *Asymptomatic, normal risk*—Individuals with no known impairment or disability and likely to be at average risk for their age and sex.
2. *Asymptomatic, high risk*—Individuals at full life activity having no present disability but aware of a measurable characteristic or asymptomatic impairment (e.g., diastolic hypertension, asthma in remission).
3. *Symptomatic*—Individuals with mild disability due to any cause (whether organic, emotional, functional, or mere anxiety) that has not disrupted their major life activity more than 20 percent of the time.
4. *Restricted*—Individuals with moderate disability such that they are restricted from their major life activity more than 25 percent of the time, but still capable of self-care activities (e.g., eating, dressing, bathing) more than 75 percent of the time.
5. *Dependent*—Individuals with severe disability and dependent on others for self-care activities more than 25 percent of the time.
6. *Dead*—Individuals for whom evidence of death can be established.

As the major levels of the scale were mutually exclusive, it was possible to augment it by additional questions to measure finer gradations of impairment or disability if this was required. Also, levels could be collapsed if necessary. In fact, Levels 1 and 2 were combined in many subsequent studies when the study team felt that it could not rely on sufficient awareness of asymptomatic impairment to distinguish those in Level 2 from those in Level 1.

The relatively simple questionnaire required by this health status scale (see Appendix A) was to be applied by a nonphysician evaluation assistant (subsequently called "health accountant") in personal or telephone interviews as well as mail surveys. First used in two studies on hypertension and myocardial infarction conducted at Baltimore City Hospitals, this procedure has become an integral part of outcome assessment studies in the health accounting project.

Estimation of Data and Priority Setting by Small Group Processes. In a longitudinal study of pediatric atopy in the state of Maryland conducted to provide a basis for the improvement of medical care to atopic children in the state (Ryan et al., 1972), an estimation of the prevalence and the natural history of pediatric atopy and of the efficacy of current treatments, as well as of costs and available resources, was undertaken to compensate for the lack of relevant research data that would provide a framework for analysis of the study findings. In the course of this project, practical methods were developed for eliciting team estimates of information needed for establishing priorities and standards for health care outcome assessment projects. These methods were subsequently tested in a feasibility study organized at the University of Leiden, in collaboration with the Philips Electric Corporation, which focused on industrial absenteeism as the main outcome of interest (Williamson and van Nieuwenhuijzen, 1974). This study sought to establish which group of employees might receive the greatest health benefit, accompanied by similar economic benefit for the corporation, if health accounting projects were to be conducted.

The nominal group judgment methods developed in these projects were subsequently applied to the task of assessment topic priority setting at the Baltimore City Hospitals. Individual estimates were elicited from provider groups regarding topics likely to encompass preventable health impairment not currently being prevented. Initial consensus was tested by having each member rate a given topic on a one to five point scale, the highest level indicating the most suitable and immediately promising topic for actual study. Individual ratings were displayed, and the topic was discussed further if a wide discrepancy in judgment was found. The team was encouraged to submit any known data to support individual judgments. After a brief discussion, in which definitional misunderstandings usually posed the major reasons for disagreement, a final scaling provided the basis for determining consensus, which in this case indicated that the major quality assurance focus at Baltimore City Hospitals should be cardiovascular disease in the emergency room population, including the topics of hypertension, heart failure, and myocardial infarction. The greatest potential for preventable impairment and disability was considered to exist in the ambulatory population with diastolic hypertension, especially in those with actual or impending heart failure. Accordingly, a prospective study was designed to assess the care provided to diastolic hypertensives seen in the hospital emergency room. Patients were followed for one year to determine whether measured health outcomes were within assessment standards formulated by the study team. A second population for care assessment was defined as all emergency room admissions complaining of chest pain and admitted to the coronary care unit for observation as acute myocardial infarction suspects. Again, special emphasis was given to the possible complication of heart failure. These patients were likewise to be followed for one year to determine whether health outcomes were within team standards (see Chapter 8 for details on these two projects).

These priority judgments proved justified in two respects. Controlled clinical trials have since confirmed the assumption by the priority setting team at Baltimore City Hospitals of efficacy of treatment (Veterans Administration Cooperative Study of Hypertension, 1972, 1970, 1967). Also, considerable preventable disability was indeed found in the study population (Williamson, 1971). It should be noted here that while estimates of efficacy of treatment may be widely applicable, estimates of performance deficiencies should as a rule not be generalized beyond the immediate scope of patient care experience of the quality assurance panel. Subsequent studies have established that the same topic can be an area of performance strength in one facility and of serious performance weakness in another.

Development of Outcome Standards. The use of nominal small group processes was extended to the development of outcome standards. In initial health accounting projects, performance standards had been implicit—e.g., all-or-none standards for laboratory test outcome studies (see Chapter 9)—or had depended upon the availability of measured norms in the literature. However, experience in the second period indicated that performance or outcome norms or average results from comparative studies are inadequate as evaluation standards. Such information, while valuable for the standard setting process, cannot substitute for facility specific standards of performance, which must reflect two elements if assessment is to result in eventual improvement:

- An estimate of what outcomes can be considered achievable given the state of the art (evidence of efficacy); and
- A judgment reflecting the extent to which that which is achievable can be achieved within the constraints of available resources and be acceptable to providers and consumers.

Because of the scarcity of efficacy data, it was recognized that expert opinion would be required to determine what outcomes are achievable. Local providers must then establish to what extent achievable benefit can be realized within the constraints of available resources, and a combination of provider and consumer judgment is necessary to provide the value judgments. What the study teams at Baltimore City Hospitals did establish in this respect was that acceptable and practical standards could be developed by teams of five or more members using formal group judgment techniques. They also provided followup data on reliability. Several months later, when standards on the same topic were elicited a second time and compared to those established earlier, it was found that although the standards set by any one panel member might vary, the team averages remained remarkably consistent.

Two broad assessment categories were given emphasis in this period: diagnostic and therapeutic outcomes, each requiring special outcome standards. Diagnostic standards were to provide the maximum acceptable percentage, among a patient group at risk, of those missed (false negative diagnoses) or invalidly included (false positive diagnoses). Therapeutic or health outcome standards were obtained by a percentage distribution of a group of patients over the previously described six level health scale, indicating maximum acceptable group disability. Failure to meet either standard would then indicate the need for further inquiry to verify deficiencies or corrective action to improve performance.

Table 6.1 illustrates two sets of standards for a study of

Table 6.1. Illustration of maximum acceptable diagnostic and therapeutic outcome standards for emergency room patients

Outcomes	*Emergency Room Patients*	
	Hypertension (complicated by heart failure)	*Heart failure in myocardial infarction suspects[b]*
Diagnostic (as percent in each category)		
False negatives (missed diagnoses)	5	5
False positives (misdiagnoses)	10	5
Therapeutic[a] (as percent at each level)		
Asymptomatic, normal and high risk	59	33
Symptomatic	18	24
Restricted	10	8
Dependent	3	13
Dead	10	22

[a] One year followup. Therapeutic outcome standards always represent a hypothetical percentage distribution over one-hundred patients.
[b] Admitted to coronary care unit.

emergency room patients at Baltimore City Hospitals; note that while the standards for false negatives were the same, the hypertension panel was prepared to accept a higher proportion of patients with erroneous diagnosis of heart failure than the panel establishing analogous standards for myocardial infarction suspects. Conversely, the outcome standard set by the hypertension panel indicated that 13 percent of such patients dependent or dead was an acceptable outcome at one year followup, whereas the standard of the myocardial infarction team accepted up to 35 percent of myocardial infarction suspects at those outcome levels. The format and methods for setting outcome assessment standards illustrated in these studies were subsequently adopted as standard procedure for nearly all health accounting projects.

The Feasibility of Health Accounting in Primary Care—1969-1973

The third period in the development of health accounting involved a large number of projects in a series of twenty multispecialty group clinics (often with their associated hospitals) throughout the United States. They were conducted to determine the feasibility of establishing multiple health accounting systems in a variety of different primary care settings and of making extensive use of salaried health accountants or evaluation assistants. A standardized procedural manual and assessment training procedures were developed. In order to obtain more detailed and reliable measurements of health care outcomes, diagnostic and therapeutic assessment categories were redefined as follows to permit the identification of specific outcomes directly related to improvement potential:

- *Case finding outcomes* indicating the level of diagnostic performance in identifying patients where improved medical care might result in substantially increased health benefits. Case finding is assessed by two measures: the false negative rate (the percentage that should have been detected but was not—i.e., missed diagnoses) and the false positive rate (the percentage that was given a specific diagnosis but should not have been so diagnosed—i.e., misdiagnoses).
- *Health problem control rates* indicating the extent to which measurable health problem outcomes permit the inference that medical control of these problems has been established (e.g., blood pressure or blood sugar control over time).
- *Overall health status outcomes* indicating the extent of group

disability in the patient sample based on the six level health status scale.

The last category, by providing an assessment measure of patient function within a social context, may be considered a proxy measure for overall patient health, crudely approximating quality of life.

Field Trials. The major practical phase of the third period was a field trial in several multispecialty group clinics to determine the feasibility of simultaneously organizing several quality assurance systems employing health accounting approaches. The setting was selected for reasons of both practicality and significance: multispecialty clinics have a sufficiently large patient population for quality assurance projects; group practice is likely to increase substantially and will become increasingly important for quality assurance in primary care; and relatively large clinics can provide the required resources and the organizational setting for practical demonstrations of assessing and improving performance. The administrative structure of group clinics was an additional incentive, as their executive boards can make formal decisions for the total group and resolve whether or not quality assurance results warrant a more substantial subsequent involvement.

Collaboration with the American Group Practice Association (formerly the American Association of Medical Clinics) was secured, and twelve clinics recommended by their executive director were contacted. These clinics had shown previous interest in quality assurance, and most of them were, or were about to be, accredited, ensuring basic standards of organization, medical record keeping, and educational activities. Eventually, partly due to endorsement by the American Group Practice Association and partly because they were interested in the health accounting project, nine of the twelve clinics agreed to participate. Eight of these were located in the Midwest and one in New England. The health accounting projects in all of these institutions were conducted under a direct collaborative arrangement between the clinics and The Johns Hopkins University, which covered the full salary of the health accountant and 10 percent of the salary of the physician appointed as quality assurance coordinator with overall responsibility for project implementation.

Subsequently, eleven more clinics joined the project. Thus, a total of twenty clinics and several affiliated hospitals constituted the research setting for the third period. In locations ranging from Massachusetts to California, they included fee for service and prepaid organizations. Four were university affiliated, eight were privately owned, and seven were members of a for profit corporation of affiliated health maintenance organizations. The respective patient populations ranged from poverty to working and middle class patients (see Chapter 7 for a detailed breakdown of both facilities and patient populations).

The reasons for project participation were usually mixed, but it is interesting to note that stated incentives included not only the desire to improve the quality of care provided to their patients and to contribute to scientific knowledge and literature in the developing field of quality assurance, but as well the expected advantages of securing new patients or panels of patients, of gaining additional financial backing, or of using personnel paid by the health accounting project for unrelated purposes.

Most of the organizational arrangements with the clinics were made either with the executive head or with the medical director with the approval of the executive head. The decision to participate was made arbitrarily by the executive head in certain cases, but discussion and approval by the medical board of these institutions was the more usual procedure. It is of interest that in nearly every instance where the decision was made in an authoritarian manner, usually by the clinic owner, participation of the staff was particularly poor, and administrative problems were multiplied. Also, though many of the clinical staff would become personally involved and participate actively, there was marked passive resistance: quality assurance tasks were given low priority; study team meetings would be put off; and members who had agreed to participate would frequently have a ready excuse for not attending. This experience demonstrates the need for more positive incentives. Throughout the total project, overall staff motivation to participate, despite the best of clinic intentions and the enthusiasm of their project staff, remained one of the most serious general administrative problems.

Another problem concerned communication. The flood of new terms and unfamiliar concepts and theories was at times overwhelming. On many occasions the clinic staff would not admit that they were totally lost, although subsequent problems with individual projects made this painfully evident. It must be admitted that in this phase of the project, the Hopkins project team were never really successful in deleting project jargon from both written or spoken communication. On the other hand, there never was a serious conflict in terms of the "town-gown" syndrome. The Hopkins team were successful in establishing a nonthreatening relationship. The project director, a nonmedical professional, was highly successful in most clinics. He was open about his lack of medical sophistication, yet firm and positive in his own understanding of health accounting. This, together with his considerable administrative abilities, facilitated the almost simultaneous implementation of this quality assurance approach in a variety of clinics. In nearly every instance, the clinic health accounting teams succeeded in completing one or more assessment studies of health care outcomes.

The health accountants hired by the clinics, who were responsible for record reviews and literature surveys, for sampling, and for patient and physician interviews, proved to be quite successful overall, despite the novelty of their role. Few complaints were received from either staff or patients. Early on there had been difficulties in a few clinics regarding staff understanding of who the health accountant was and why he was given so much latitude in and about the clinic. Institutional cues, such as white coats, nametags, and printed personal name cards, together with formal introductions in staff meetings to physicians and nonphysician personnel, usually solved such problems. Understanding and backing by the clinic power structure, however, was the single most important prerequisite to success. Without this, some health accountants had difficulty securing even a desk at which to work, much less active cooperation.

Assessing Administrative and Fiscal Outcomes of Care. In the latter half of Period Three, an effort was made to explore methods for assessing aspects of efficiency by extending and modifying health accounting principles developed for the assessment and improvement of effectiveness of care. In view of increasing concerns over costs, this seemed a fruitful direction to take. Seven prepaid clinics who were members of a for profit corporation franchising and managing health maintenance organizations agreed to participate in this effort, and there was considerable interest in this undertaking by the corporation. However, when the appointed team (representing all participating clinics) met to conduct the priority setting meeting, most of the topics selected appeared to relate to care effectiveness rather than to care efficiency, despite considerable effort to encourage focus on the business and administrative side. So as not to let the project flounder, this change of emphasis was accepted on the understanding that financial aspects would at least be ancillary topics and become a major focus later. However, even this limited effort proved so unsuccessful that the economic aspects of the studies have only been briefly mentioned in the data presented in Chapters 8-10. A major difficulty was to obtain unit cost data related to patients categorized by diagnosis. This lack of useful cost data is well known and has been described frequently (Sorensen, 1976).

The benefit of hindsight would indicate that such efficiency projects require professionals with backgrounds in finance and economics and with experience with cost benefit or cost effectiveness analyses in health care. However, there is no intrinsic reason, given sufficient input from management and more focused guidance, why health accounting methods of deductive outcome assessment and improvement cannot be applied to the assessment and improvement of care efficiency as well.

THE STRUCTURE OF A HEALTH ACCOUNTING SYSTEM: ORGANIZATION AND FUNCTION

As the ultimate purpose of health accounting is the development and implementation of a practicable management resource for health care assessment and improvement, the health accounting system is based on a series of procedures that are common to all projects but permit a wide range of both assessment and improvement topics and methods. The basic components involve:

- A common administrative structure including a quality assurance executive board, a quality assurance coordinator who is a staff physician, and an evaluation assistant (i.e., the health accountant);
- Systematic assessment of care outcomes, with focus on priority topics judged by local staff to have the greatest potential for improving effectiveness and/or efficiency of performance within acceptable limits of effort;
- A range of outcome as well as other assessment methods for identifying correctable determinants of outcome deficiencies;
- A cyclic project design consisting of identifying deficiencies, implementing actions to achieve improvement, assessing the results, and taking whatever subsequent actions are required to obtain further improvement;
- Successively more detailed group estimations of the likely costs and benefits (especially health benefits) to be derived from further effort on a particular topic.

The group commitment implicit in this structure is intended to promote active staff interest and inquiry into aspects such as the improvement of estimates of achievable benefit and to increase the impact of assessment in terms of documented improvement in performance, especially as related to patient health.

The Organization of Health Accounting at the Project Site

The administrative structure of health accounting systems as it evolved over the first ten years (1963-1973) has provided an adaptable framework for the 56 health accounting projects described in Chapters 7-10 and a subsequent series of 18 projects. By 1973, the administrative structure at the project sites, including university medical centers, community hospitals, corporate clinics, and private group clinics, was constituted as follows (see also Figure 6.2):

The quality assurance executive board;
The quality assurance coordinator;
The health accountant;
The priority team; and
The study teams.

The Quality Assurance Executive Board. The quality assurance executive board was recognized as an essential component on the basis of the experience gathered during the initial stages of health accounting (1963-1969). In early studies, it had been noted that quality assurance efforts were usually confined to a small group of

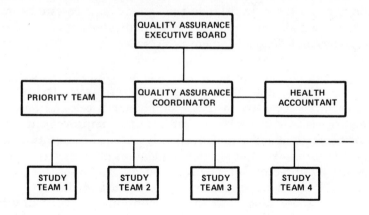

Figure 6.2. The administrative structure of a health accounting project at the project site.

interested participants and often had little or no impact outside that group. Since an essential principle of health accounting is that it must be an integral part of the clinic or hospital management system and play a role analogous to that of financial accounting, the executive board, as the core power structure of the institution, would have to assume responsibility for comparing costs and benefits of quality assurance activity as well as for policy formulation and executive management. Without decisional incorporation into the power structure, quality assurance studies will remain isolated endeavors of little value.

The quality assurance executive board is thus essential because it represents the decision making bodies of the institution. It has the authority to allocate resources and to authorize the hiring of new personnel, the purchasing of new equipment, and the reorganization of operations within the institution. In health accounting, the board makes the final selection of topics for assessment study and judges whether identified deficiencies seem serious enough to warrant further correction. The board approves plans for improvement, including any expenditures required to improve effectiveness or efficiency. It also decides when to stop further effort on any topic and when to move on to a new project on the priority list.

The Quality Assurance Coordinator. From the beginning, the quality assurance coordinator has been an important personnel resource. As shown by the experience of the many health accounting projects, a respected physician can fill this role successfully. If the quality assurance executive board sets policy, the quality assurance coordinator must see to it that this policy is successfully implemented, evaluated, and reported back to the board. Also, in most of the clinics and hospitals where health accounting has been implemented, there usually were multiple concurrent assessment and improvements functions. Most already had utilization review groups, tissue committees, and death committees (especially the hospitals involved); more recently, medical audit committees had been constituted to evaluate the care provided. Often, improvement actions were being recommended independently of such monitoring mechanisms, for example, in continuing education programs as routinely conducted by directors of medical education. To be successfully implemented, a health accounting system must obviously be coordinated with these other activities. A coordinator aware of all ongoing quality assurance activities is an important liaison to the executive board, in addition to integrating the work of the study teams within the health accounting system, who may be focusing on multiple and concomitant quality assurance topics. Instances where the study teams were organized independently by interested staff made it clear that a single coordinator with authority above these teams was essential to avoid conflicts and wasted effort. There has been little or no question in most quality assurance systems in or out of health accounting regarding the need for a single executive leader. In most of the health accounting projects reported here, the quality assurance coordinator was a physician with interest in quality assurance who was trained by the Johns Hopkins project personnel to organize the priority team and the individual study teams. The coordinator usually sits with the executive board and transmits results from and conveys the board's instructions to the teams. He facilitates continuity and coordination with other quality assurance activities in the organization, including continuing medical education, which collectively take up considerable time in any institution and thus require decisions as to relative priorities.

The Health Accountant. The central role of the health accountant in the routine but time consuming task of assessment data collection, including literature reviews and prevalence checks of specific health problems, is now well established. Earlier, these tasks had been done by postgraduate physicians, residents, and medical students, but it was quickly realized that most required very little, if any, medical expertise. Thus, health accountants are now non-physicians, such as nurses or technicians, or undergraduate students and sometimes come from outside the health field, although some data management or research experience is essential. Hired to assist in conducting the quality assurance activities of the facility, their major functions are gathering information, whether from the literature, medical records, or patient interview and followup; assisting quality assurance team members when needed; and writing reports and documenting activities and results.

The Priority Team. The establishment of priority teams and the formalization of the process for identifying priority topics for quality assurance study is one of the most important features of health accounting. Originally, most topics had been selected by the quality assurance coordinator, with informal consultation provided by staff members and occasional evaluative input by the Johns Hopkins project staff. The quality of these topics was usually mixed, and the motivations and criteria for topic nomination and selection were varied. More importantly, the value of project findings was often nil as regarded improvement of care, let alone patient health.

In retrospect, the physicians would usually admit freely that they had consciously selected topics that would make them "look good" or for which findings could be assembled quickly and simply regardless of their subsequent value for the improvement of outcomes of care in their facilities. In other words, by the physicians' own admission, most project failures in terms of their inability to identify serious but remediable care deficiencies could have been predicted before the project was implemented.

Another problem encountered was the understandable propensity of most clinicians to characterize problems for study by traditional health problems, as reflected in the frequent selection of diabetes, hypertension, or urinary tract infections as study topics. To overcome this limitation, the concept of achievable health benefits not achieved (see Chapter 3) was stressed as the overriding principle in quality assurance topic selection. To apply this concept, a formal priority team is convened and given a training session in the task of establishing quality assurance topic priorities. The team is first taught to establish and quantify achievable health benefits and to recognize that the extent of such benefits is defined by the validity of evidence of current diagnostic and therapeutic efficacy. Furthermore, such benefits must be quantified in terms of benefit per person times the number of persons involved; in other words, slight benefit per person times a large number of people may equal extensive benefit per person times a small number of people.

Next, the team must judge to what extent the benefit found achievable is in fact not presently being achieved by the care provided. This aspect of team judgment forces careful consideration and priority setting in regard to care deficiencies possibly occurring at present. The final consideration is the feasibility of conducting a study of the topic selected and the probability of effecting genuine improvement in view of the team's knowledge of time and resource limitations as well as of the limitations inherent in efforts at effecting behavioral change.

Eventually, the priority team evolved as a group of seven to eleven persons representing major aspects of an institution's health care operations. It consists of several physicians and a nurse, administrator, technician, and physician assistant; where indicated, technical or front desk personnel may be included. It meets only twice—once for training and once to establish topic priorities for quality assurance projects. This group must take a comprehensive view of the operations of its institution and identify those areas where correctable deficiencies directly related to unacceptable health outcomes (aspects of effectiveness) or unacceptable expenditures in time, money, or other resources (aspects of efficiency) may exist. Topics suggested must be analyzed in terms of assessment cost effectiveness. Subsequent tests of priority team functions have documented the reliability and validity of this procedure in multispecialty group clinics (Williamson et al., 1977; Horn and Williamson, 1977) and have confirmed provider judgment in identifying potential for improvement in local health care outcomes (Williamson, Braswell and Horn, 1978).

The Study Team. The study teams implement the individual assessment studies. When the quality assurance executive board authorizes a project, a group representing specialists from the topic area is appointed. Study teams generally have five members, and if the topic is medical, the team usually has two to three physicians; if the topic is administrative in nature, only one or two may be necessary. It is important that the group include persons who are most familiar with the topic, as they are able to define the problem in sufficient detail to make assessment possible. The team defines a sampling frame and sampling method, develops outcome standards and measures for assessment, and provides explicit estimates of the health benefits to be achieved or of unnecessary expenditures of resources to be saved by implementing the proposed project. This information represents the third and most definitive estimate of cost effectiveness of quality assurance activity on the topic, the first having been made by the priority team and the second by the quality assurance board in authorizing the study. Assessment details are designed in one or two meetings. The health accountant then pretests the instruments recommended and, if they are successful, is authorized to carry out the study. The team meets again to analyze the results and to make recommendations to the quality assurance board regarding further action for effective improvement if a serious deficiency is uncovered. The team dissolves once improvement is achieved, future assessment monitoring scheduled, or further action in the topic area considered inadvisable.

Summary: The Functional Stages of a Health Accounting Project

Health accounting has evolved into a five stage cyclic strategy (see Figure 6.3) designed to improve health care outcomes. Diagnostic and therapeutic outcomes were stressed in the first ten years of health accounting, but procedures that analyze the cost effectiveness and organizational impact of a project can be conducted prospectively, in conjunction with the various stages of the project (Williamson et al., 1975).

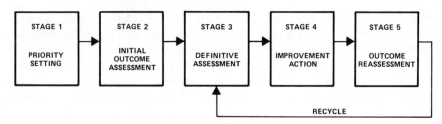

Figure 6.3. The health accounting strategy: a five stage approach to improvement of care.

In Stage 1, topics for assessment and improvement are selected by a priority setting mechanism, whereby a team of qualified medical and other health personnel familiar with the clinic or hospital (or any other health care setting) determine, by small group estimation techniques, those aspects of care or administration in their facility where change might result in substantial health improvement or cost reduction (Williamson, 1978). These potential quality assurance topics encompass the achievable benefit not presently being achieved (see Chapter 3), whether in regard to specific health problems that are not being correctly diagnosed or managed, health outcomes for patient groups, or administrative and organizational problems such as the timeliness and appropriateness of scheduled appointments. A wide range of problems can thus be addressed in health accounting, since this approach is not exclusively dependent on information sources such as medical records but can obtain the required data for assessment by independent encounter forms and other relatively simple means.

In Stage 2, deficiencies are identified by initial outcome assessment. This assessment is designed by a second team of qualified staff members of the clinic, sometimes with the aid of an outside specialist in a field relevant to the topic to be studied. An assessment design is developed incorporating explicit estimates of the total potential gain in the target benefit that can be achieved at that facility. These estimates provide a basis for predicting the potential impact of the study; they also provide standards for evaluating the outcome. Measures of diagnostic and therapeutic outcomes are obtained by the health accountant, and measured results are then compared with the standards previously established by the team. If serious discrepancies are found, further action in the subsequent stages of the strategy is usually recommended.

Stage 3 encompasses a more definitive assessment of the causes of the deficient outcomes determined in Stage 2. Again, the design is provided by staff members on the study team, and the measures are made by the health accountant. Where correctable outcomes can be identified, improvement action is planned.

In Stage 4, improvement actions are implemented (e.g., various educational or administrative measures).

In Stage 5, verification of improvement is undertaken by means of a replication of the original assessment of results to determine whether standards have now been met. If the standards set in Stage 2 have not been met, Stages 3, 4, and 5 are repeated one or more times either until acceptable improvement has been achieved or until it becomes apparent that any subsequent gain will not be worth the further effort required.

REFERENCES

Dryer, B.V. 1962. Lifetime learning for physicians: principles, practices, proposals. *J Med Educ* 37(6) pt. 2.

Ellwood, P.; O'Donoghue, P.; and McClure, W. 1973. *Assuring the Quality of Care.* Minneapolis: Interstudy.

Emlet, H.E.; Williamson, J.W.; Dittmer, D.L.; and Davis, J.L. 1973. *Estimated Health Benefits and Cost of Post-Onset Care for Stroke in a Three-State Area: Minnesota, North Dakota, and South Dakota.* Falls Church, Va.: Analytic Services.

Gonnella, J.S., Goran, M.J.; Williamson, J.W.; and Cotsonas, W.J. 1970. Evaluation of patient care—an approach. *JAMA* 214:2040-43.

Horn, S.D., and Williamson, J.W. 1977. Statistical methods for reliability and validity testing: an application to nominal group judgments in health care. *Med Care* 15:922-28.

Ryan, M.B.; Nathanson, C.A.; Mellits, D.E.; and Rodman, A.C. 1972. *Determination of the Prevalence and Special Needs of Children with Bronchial Asthma or Atopic Dermatitis.* Final Report for the Department of Health, Education and Welfare, Children's Bureau, Project Nos. 212 and H-188(R). Baltimore: The Johns Hopkins University.

Sorensen, J.E. 1976. Uniform cost accounting in long-term care. In *Long-Term Care Data. Report on the Conference on Long-Term Health Care Data,* J. Murnaghan, ed., pp. 154-59. Philadelphia: Lippincott. Reprinted from *Med Care* (14)5 Supplement.

Storey, P.B.; Williamson, J.W.; and Castle, C.H. 1968. *Continuing Medical Education—A New Emphasis.* Chicago: American Medical Association.

Veterans Administration Cooperative Study Group on Antihypertensive Agents. 1967. Effects of treatment on morbidity in hypertension. Results for patients with diastolic blood pressure averaging 115 through 129 mm Hg. *JAMA* 202:1028-34.

———. 1970. Effects of treatment on morbidity in hypertension, pt. 2: Results in patients with diastolic blood pressure averaging 90 through 114 mm Hg. *JAMA* 213:1143-52.

——. 1972. Effects of treatment on morbidity in hypertension, pt. 3: Influence of age, diastolic pressure and prior cardiovascular disease; further analysis of side-effects. *Circulation* 45:991-1004.

Williamson, J.W. 1962. A Problem in Continuing Medical Education of Practicing Physicians—A Report submitted to the American Heart Association in application for a Research Fellowship.

——. 1971. Evaluating the quality of patient care—a strategy relating outcome and process assessment. *JAMA* 218:564-69.

——. 1978. Formulating priorities for quality assurance activity—description of a method and its application. *JAMA* 239:631-37.

Williamson, J.W.; Alexander, M.; and Miller, G.E. 1967. Continuing education and patient care research—physician response to screening test results. *JAMA* 201:938-42.

——. 1968. Priorities in patient care research and continuing medical education. *JAMA* 204:93-98.

Williamson, J.W.; Aronovitch, S.; Simonson, L.; Ramirez, C.; and Kelly, D. 1975. Health accounting: an outcome based system of quality assurance: illustrative application to hypertension. *Bull NY Acad Med* 51:727-38.

Williamson, J.W.; Braswell, H.R.; and Horn, S.D. 1978. Validity of staff judgments in establishing quality assurance priorities. *Med Care* (in press).

Williamson, J.W.; Braswell, H.R.; Horn, S.D.; and Lohmeyer, S. 1978. Priority setting in quality assurance: reliability of staff judgment in medical institutions. *Med Care* (in press).

Williamson, J.W.; Horn, S.D.; Choi, T.; and White, P.E. 1977. Evaluating an outcome-based quality assurance system. Final Project Report, Grant 5-R01-HS01590, National Center for Health Services Research, Department of Health, Education and Welfare. Baltimore: The Johns Hopkins School of Hygiene and Public Health (processed).

Williamson, J.W., and van Nieuwenhuijzen, M.G. 1974. Health benefit analysis—an application in industrial absenteeism. *J Occup Med* 16:229-33.

Chapter 7

An Overview of Health Accounting Projects and Results

During the first ten years of health accounting (1963–1973), 59 quality assurance projects were designed, of which 57 were implemented and 56 completed. These encompassed a total of 88 separate assessment studies, as many projects conducted different types of assessment for the same health problem topic and sample population. Details on the design and implementation of these projects and on the assessment findings will be reported in Chapters 8–10; the following provides a brief overview of the participating facilities, sampling methods, completion rates, assessment topics, and specific procedures used.

A SUMMARY OF HEALTH ACCOUNTING PROJECTS: 1963–1973

Provider and Patient Characteristics

Facilities and Physicians. Table 7.1 shows the type, financing mechanism, and location of the facilities involved in the first ten years of health accounting. The 23 facilities comprised university medical centers, including university managed outpatient and community clinics (6), community hospitals (2), corporate health maintenance organizations (7), and private group ambulatory clinics (8). Five projects were located in hospitals or in clinics associated with hospitals. The customary method of payment for services was fee for service in 9 facilities, prepaid in 11 facilities, and mixed in 3 facilities. Physician staff consisted of specialists to a large extent; most primary

Table 7.1. Health accounting facilities by type, financing mechanism, and location in the United States, 1963-1973

Facility Type	Financing Mechanism			Location in United States		
	Prepaid	Fee for service	Mixed	East	Central	West
University medical centers[a]	3	3		4	2	
Community hospitals	1	1		1	1	
Corporate clinics (HMO)	7					7
Private group clinics		5	3	3	5	
Total	11	9	3	8	8	7

[a]Includes university managed outpatient and community clinics.

care was given by general internists and pediatricians. Geographic location ranged from Massachusetts to California, with almost equal concentration in the eastern (8), central (8), and western (7) parts of the country. Except for the borderline states of Kentucky and Maryland, the southern United States was not represented.

In general, therefore, an overall balance of facilities with regard to size, method of payment, and location can be observed. However, there were some significant gaps, particularly the lack of involvement of solo practitioners and a notable scarcity of general practitioners. This exclusion of an important segment of primary ambulatory care was due to practical constraints, but it may tend to bias the results obtained and to restrict the general applicability of conclusions concerning the effectiveness of health accounting in primary care. As pointed out in Chapter 4, although solo practitioners account for the largest single provider group in medical care, they have been generally neglected in assessment of care studies because of difficulties in identifying and sampling the patients for whom the practitioner has major responsibility, in finding sufficient numbers of patients with specified health problems whose care could be assessed, and in obtaining sufficient information from office medical records. The preponderance of specialists in most of the studies reported here may be another bias. There is evidence that general practitioners find it slightly more difficult to participate meaningfully in quality assessment studies (Peterson et al., 1956; Clute, 1963; Payne et al., 1976). It may well be, therefore, that the success in obtaining the cooperation of physicians in the projects reported may relate to this biased selection of providers.

Patient Characteristics. Table 7.2 summarizes selected characteristics of the patient populations of the facilities participating in

Table 7.2. Selected characteristics of patient populations served by twenty-three facilities conducting health accounting studies, 1963–1973

| | Patient Population Characteristics | | | | | | | | | | |
| | Community type | | | | Predominant socioeconomic class served by facility | | | | Predominant method of payment | | |
Community Size	Urban	Rural	Sub-urban	Urban/ rural	Middle	Working	Poverty	Mixed	Private insur-ance	Insur-ance/ cash	Medicare/ Medicaid or welfare
More than 1 million	7						4	3		2	5
100,000 to 1 million	7		1			2	2	4		5	3
Less than 100,000	1	4	1	2	1	3	1	3	1	6	1
Total	15	4	2	2	1	5	7	10	1	13	9

the study. Seven clinics were located in large populations centers (>1,000,000), 8 in medium-sized (between 100,000 and 1,000,000) and another 8 in small population centers (<100,000). Urban centers predominated (15); the remainder were divided between suburban (2), rural (4), and mixed urban/rural areas (2). The predominance of urban locations may mean that community health resources such as emergency transportation and tertiary care were relatively accessible to the patient population.

The predominant socioeconomic classes served were as follows: middle class, 1 facility; working class, 5 facilities; predominantly poverty class, 7 facilities, and mixed (usually middle and working and working and poverty class), 10 facilities. As minority or poverty group patients predominated in 7 settings, among them 4 facilities in the large population centers, patients on welfare were overrepresented in these studies, most likely due to the relatively large number of university or university affiliated medical centers (6) among the participating institutions. Although followup of patients in this socioeconomic group is generally considered difficult, this was not supported by the response rates obtained (see also Table 7.4).

Private insurance or cash payments were the predominant source of payment in 14 facilities; Medicare/Medicaid or welfare predominated in the remaining 9 facilities.

Sampling and Survey Results

With regard to the sampling and survey results of the 1963–1973 phase of health accounting, it should be noted that they were obtained by clinic or hospital teams who, for the most part, were inexperienced in survey research. Of the 57 projects implemented, 38 used a retrospective consecutive sample, going back in time until an adequate sample size was obtained; 16 used a prospective consecutive sample, listing appropriate walk-in patients until a sufficient number was collected; 2 studies used a probability sampling method; and one study was discontinued. Of the completed projects, 18 used clinic charts as a sampling base; 13, consecutive walk-in patients; 1, consecutive new clinic admissions; 5, clinic computer records; 7, patient hospital charts; 2, consecutive hospital or coronary care unit admissions; and 5, hospital or clinic laboratory test reports. Surgical reports were used in 4 studies, and in one study the sampling base was not specified.

Of the 56 completed projects, 26 involved assessment of diagnostic outcomes (misdiagnoses and missed diagnoses), covering an aggregate of 15,163 patients. Of these 26 projects, 23 involved chart review

Table 7.3. Aggregate final samples and completion rates in diagnostic and therapeutic outcome projects, 1963–1973

Outcome Category	Number of Projects	Patients Sampled	Number of Patients with Complete Outcome Data	Aggregate Completion Rate (percent)
Diagnostic	26	15,163[a]	14,165	93.4
Therapeutic	47[b]	6,150	4,900	79.7
Direct followup studies	44	5,943[c]	4,767	80.2
Chart review only	2	207	133	64.3

[a]Excluding Study 45, where denominator data were insufficient for determination of completion rates.
[b]Study 4 used both direct followup and chart review methods.
[c]Excluding Study 6, where denominator data were insufficient for determination of completion rates.

and 3 applied direct patient measurements. Complete diagnostic outcome measurements were obtained for 14,165 of the 15,163 patients sampled, for an aggregate completion rate of 93.4 percent, as shown in Table 7.3. Therapeutic outcomes (health problem status and health and functional levels) were assessed in 47 studies covering an aggregate of 6,150 patients. Of these projects, 44 measured health status by means of direct patient followup, 2 involved retrospective chart review only, and 1 used both designs. Complete outcome data were obtained for 4,900 patients of the 6,150 sampled, for an aggregate completion rate of 79.7 percent. A further breakdown of these data revealed that among the 45 prospective or direct followup studies, complete data were obtained from 4,767 of the 5,943 patients sampled, yielding an aggregate response rate of 80.2 percent for projects involving prospective data collection (see Table 7.3).

An overview of sample sizes and completion rates by socioeconomic characteristics of the patient populations is provided in Table 7.4. For diagnostic outcome assessment, which was mainly based on chart review, the highest completion rates were obtained for predominantly poverty populations (96.2 percent), followed closely by mixed working/middle class and poverty/working class populations (94.2 percent and 92.6 percent), with working class patients lowest (84.3 percent); it is interesting to note that there were no diagnostic outcome studies conducted in facilities serving middle class populations exclusively. In the therapeutic outcome studies, which on the whole used direct followup of patients or prospective methods, the

Table 7.4. Patient samples and completion rates in twenty-three health accounting facilities, by socioeconomic patient characteristics

Socioeconomic Patient Characteristics[a]	Number of Facilities	Number of Projects in these Facilities	Diagnostic Outcome Assessment			Therapeutic Outcome Assessment		
			Total patients sampled	Complete patient data obtained (n)	Completion rate (percent)	Total patients sampled	Complete patient data obtained (n)	Completion rate (percent)
Poverty	7	12	5,342	5,138	96.2	1,302	956	73.4
Poverty and working	2	2	122	113	92.6	194	185	95.4
Working	5	13	2,274	1,917	84.3	1,613	1,485	92.1
Working and middle	8	25	7,425	6,997	94.2	2,617	1,941	74.2
Middle	1	4	0	0	--	424	333	78.5
Total	23	56	15,163	14,165	93.4	6,150	4,900	79.7

[a]Predominant group served by facility as stated by facility staff.
--Not applicable.

highest completion rates were achieved for mixed poverty and working class populations (95.4 percent), followed by working class (92.1 percent), middle class (78.5 percent), and mixed working/middle class populations (74.2 percent), with the poverty class completion rate slightly lower (73.4 percent).

The feasibility of the health accounting approach is, therefore, at least partly indicated by the generally adequate response rates obtained. This proved true in terms both of retrospective chart data collection for diagnostic outcome assessment (93.4 percent completion rate overall) and of prospective patient followup for therapeutic outcome assessment (79.7 percent completion rate overall). It was particularly encouraging to note that it was possible to instruct clinic personnel inexperienced in survey research in procedures that yielded an overall completion rate of 89.5 percent. This would seem to indicate both successful planning and a great amount of willingness on the part of the patients who cooperated in these studies. This finding is probably one of the more important results of the early health accounting experience. In particular, the completion rates for direct patient followup among all social classes included in the projects strongly suggest that it is possible to break away from traditional chart audits and directly assess health outcomes in meaningful prospective studies. Even the somewhat lower overall poverty class completion rates were due largely to relatively poor results in two of the seven clinics conducting followup investigations of patients in this socioeconomic group. This is in contrast to three clinics surveying similar populations that, with moderate effort, were able to achieve high response rates (82, 92, and 92 percent, respectively).

Summary of Assessment Topics and Health Problem Focus

Of the 56 completed projects, 18 focused on both diagnostic and therapeutic outcomes, 9 solely on diagnostic outcomes, and 29 solely on therapeutic outcomes. Of the diagnostic outcome studies, 14 assessed false negative or missed diagnoses and 2 false positive or misdiagnoses exclusively, and 11 assessed both diagnostic outcome types, for a total of 13 false positive and 25 false negative diagnostic assessments (see Table 7.5). Therapeutic outcome assessment topics predominated because such studies were considered less complex and more directly related to health outcomes and therefore more suitable for demonstration projects. Experience has shown, however, that it is better to combine both from the beginning to provide a check on the success of physicians in identifying patients where therapeutic assessment is essential.

Table 7.5. Number of diagnostic and therapeutic outcome assessment studies by assessment focus and health problem

Outcome Assessed	Hypertension and Ulcer	Infectious Disease	Endocrine Disease	Neoplastic Disease	Cardiovascular-Cerebrovascular Disease	Fractures
False positives[a]	2	4	1	0	1	0
False negatives[b]	8	6	2	0	1	0
Health status	10	6	3	4	4	0
Health problem	0	2	0	0	0	2
Total	20	18	6	4	6	2

[a]Misdiagnoses.

[b]Missed diagnoses.

[c]Differences between observed findings and maximum acceptable standards were significant at $P < 0.05$ levels or better, except for Study 6, where the difference was accepted as significant at $P < 0.1$ level.

Note: Study 33, establishing patient satisfaction with care received, is not included in this count as no assessment standards were developed.

Of 87 completed studies, 50 were successful in identifying statistically significant outcome deficiencies, 32 applied formal analysis procedures to determine causes of detected deficiencies, and 30 identified correctable determinants of the outcome deficiencies established. Of this group, 23 resulted in plans for improvement action, and in 18 of these, the plans were implemented. Finally, in this last group, 15 were reevaluated and 8 were found to have succeeded in achieving improvement. In terms of overall quality assurance results, therefore, it is evident that while most of the studies succeeded in identifying serious outcome deficiencies, few attempted to achieve change and even fewer succeeded. This underscores the need for a more detailed understanding of why so little improvement action is taken even when apparently serious health care deficiencies are found.

The fact, for example, that some clinic staffs could identify as many as 48 percent of their hypertensive patients as being out of control but were not motivated to take corrective action illustrates a

Surgery	Lab Tests	Prenatal Screening	Psychiatry	Family Planning	Total	Statistically Significant Outcome Deficiencies[c]	
						n	%
0	2	0	1	1	13	5	42
0	6	1	1	1	25	22	85
5	2	0	4	1	39	20	51
2	0	1	3	0	10	3	30
7	10	2	9	3	87	50	57

not uncommon finding in these early studies. On subsequent inquiry, few of the provider groups questioned the validity of the deficient outcomes when they examined the study data in detail. The most frequent reason given, however, was the fact that "they were too busy" to attend to such "project activity." This may indicate that physicians considered these projects somehow not related to their practice. It may also indicate that their present concern for providing "care," however deficient, takes precedence over concern for the subsequent health of their patients. Indeed, the concern for "productivity" in terms of getting the patients through the system may have serious consequences in terms of ultimate health outcome. Results of replicated controlled clinical trials involving detection and treatment of hypertension indicate that a substantial proportion of present strokes and incidents of heart failure might have been prevented if physicians had been more concerned with blood pressure control of their patients. On the other hand, the health accounting projects described were successful in identifying serious care deficiencies having direct influence on patient health outcomes.

METHODS OF DATA COLLECTION AND ANALYSIS

Assessment Study Design

Sampling and Data Collection. The range of patient sampling plans employed in these outcome assessment studies is an important aspect for understanding the implications of the findings and the universe to which they can be generalized. Both retrospective and prospective sampling designs were used, the samples being identified either from listings such as medical charts, tumor registers, laboratory slips, or administrative records or from consecutive hospital admissions or walk-in patients upon first or followup contact with the clinic or hospital. Some studies used patient information that was available from existing sources; in others, direct patient followup provided the basis for assessment measures. Most projects combined these two methods, data for diagnostic outcome assessment usually being collected retrospectively, and data for therapeutic outcomes in almost all cases being obtained prospectively.

For purposes of assessment and analysis, the study population in each case was constituted by the group of measurable sampling units that represented the universe from which the population at risk and the final study sample were drawn. Both people and paper sources were used to define the study population, depending on whether prospective sampling by patient interviews or retrospective sampling by the review of clinical records was indicated to identify the population at risk and the sample. Frames for prospective sampling included consecutive annual new enrollees or clinic admissions (initial visits), or consecutive hospital admissions, clinic visits (initial and followup), and clinic contacts (telephone calls and visits). Retrospective sampling frames were constituted by total prepaid plan enrollment files, medical record files, surgery or tumor registers, laboratory or radiology test files, and administrative files.

These study populations were considered subsets of a theoretical total hospital or clinic population that cannot be enumerated for any practical purpose (Densen, 1972). A subsample comprising the population at risk for the health problem or intervention that is the assessment focus and from which the study sample can be obtained must thus be defined. Any single characteristic or combination of characteristics can be stipulated for identifying such a population subset, and depending on the study design, this subset can be either at the same risk as the parent group or at higher risk. The first type of subset is obtained by a random or consecutive selection, e.g., a brief time sample of an annual patient population (every third walk-in patient in one month), or a consecutive subsample of records (every tenth record in the file). More selective factors are used to identify a population subset at greater risk for a given health problem, e.g., demographic characteristics (all males over 65 for a study of prostatic hypertrophy) or clinical symptoms, signs, or laboratory test results (all patients receiving a chest x-ray or having "pneumonia" recorded on the radiology report in a study of pneumonia). From this population at risk, a further subset is identified as the study sample, i.e., that subset of (or occasionally the total) population at risk to which final outcome assessment measures will be applied for quality assurance purposes.

In the outcome assessment stage, the study sample is divided into three different, though overlapping, subgroups to form the following denominator groups:

- *Diagnostic Denominator 1* is that subset of the study sample that requires (1) a given diagnostic screening procedure, (2) a given diagnostic label, or (3) a given therapeutic intervention or alteration of treatment. This is the denominator for calculating the percentage of false negatives and consists of the sum of all true positives and false negatives in the study sample.
- *Diagnostic Denominator 2* is that subset of the study sample that received (1) a given diagnostic screening procedure, (2) a given diagnostic screening label, or (3) a given therapeutic intervention or alteration of treatment. This is the denominator for calculating the percentage of false positives and consists of the sum of all true positives and false positives in the study sample.
- *The Therapeutic Denominator* is that subset of the study sample followed to measure overall health status or health problem outcomes, whether constituted by the Denominator 1 or 2 group or the entire study sample.

The interrelationship of these outcome assessment sampling populations is illustrated in Figure 7.1.

Outcome Measures. In the quality assurance projects reported in Chapters 8-10, both diagnostic (case finding) outcomes and therapeutic (health) outcomes were measured.

Diagnostic (Case Finding) Outcomes. Diagnostic outcomes provide assessment measures of provider performance in identifying or excluding patients from the group to be studied for quality assurance

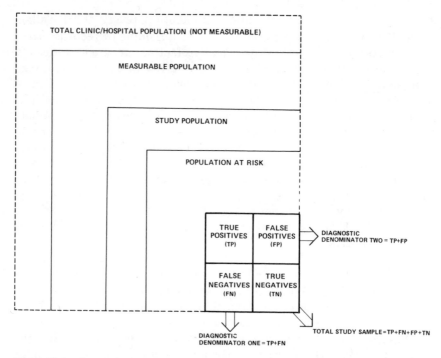

Figure 7.1. Interrelationship of outcome assessment sample populations, where Diagnostic Denominator 1 is the sum of true positives and false negatives (intervention required) and Diagnostic Denominator 2 is the sum of true positives and false positives (intervention received), and where the study sample is the sum of all four diagnostic categories. The therapeutic denominator can be either or both of the diagnostic denominators.

purposes. They are stated as percentages of false negatives (missed diagnoses) and of false positives (misdiagnoses) for the diagnostic denominator groups and fall into the following three categories:

Diagnostic screening outcomes are assessed to measure the accuracy with which patients at risk are identified. For example, of new clinic admissions with one or more indications of possible urinary tract infection (e.g., a history of chronic pyelonephritis, recent urological surgery, or a positive routine testuria laboratory test), how many patients were so identified by the clinic staff? False negatives here are those patients who were proven by independent assessment study to have had such indications but who were not identified as such, as shown by recorded staff notes, subsequent interventions, or personal inquiry of the physician. False positives are patients not having any of the above indications but who were erroneously identified as being at risk (e.g., cystitis recorded in the medical chart when the patient actually had cervicitis).

Generic diagnostic outcomes are measured by the accuracy with which patients who actually have a given health problem—as opposed to merely being suspected or at risk—are identified and labeled. Of patients having one or more indications for possible urinary tract infection (e.g., recent pregnancy), how many do in fact have such a problem? Again, false negatives are patients with subsequently verified definitive evidence of the health problem but no positive diagnosis, and false positives are those diagnosed as having the problem although, according to available data, the diagnosis was not warranted (an invalid diagnosis of urinary tract infection due to a laboratory error in reporting urine culture results).

Treatment evaluation outcomes are measured by the accuracy with which patients requiring a specific therapeutic intervention or alteration of treatment are identified. False negatives in this category refer to patients requiring but not receiving a given therapy and false positives to those who received but did not require it. Of those patients requiring a hysterectomy, how many are so identified? Of those patients receiving a hysterectomy, how many did not require it? This category applies to patients who have been screened for initial problem detection, for whom a generic diagnosis has been made, and where the major management objective is health problem control.

In Table 7.6, hypertension patients as a group provide an example of these three classes of diagnostic outcome measurement, the distinction between which is important to recognize. Though the term "diagnostic outcomes" is accurate, it is frequently interpreted within the narrow confines of the traditional concept of definitive health problem labeling. Use of the term "case finding" might be preferable to indicate the much broader range of circumstances where measures of diagnostic false negatives and false positives apply.

Therapeutic (Health) Outcomes. Therapeutic outcomes usually refer to patient health results, either in terms of treatment provided or of treatment required but omitted. Here, *health problem control outcomes* are assessed to measure the achievement of providers in controlling or preventing symptoms or specific impairments but do not include overall patient health status and functional disability. These are the outcomes most familiar to practitioners, usually involving isolated problems at the level of cells, organs, and organ systems. However, this outcome class can also encompass general problems such as fatigue or depression, specific interpersonal

Table 7.6.   Examples of three diagnostic outcome categories for quality of care assessment

Category	Measured Outcomes[a] (percent)
Diagnostic screening	
False negatives—Patients with isolated high blood pressure reading who are not subsequently screened	64
False positives—Patients given an extensive but unwarranted screening evaluation for secondary hypertension (only one elevated blood pressure recorded in the chart among normal readings)	6
Generic diagnosis	
False negatives—Hypertension patients with a correctable cause (renal artery stenosis) that is not detected	3
False positives—Essential hypertension patients erroneously diagnosed as having correctable cause	6
Treatment evaluation	
False negatives—Hypertension patients with toxic reaction to medication undetected by their physician	6
False positives—Hypertension patients with symptoms erroneously attributed to antihypertensive medication	15

[a]The percent of false negatives and false positives do not add, as they are computed from different denominators.

problems such as sexual maladjustment or child abuse, or even specific social problems such as delinquency or occupational or family maladjustment that involve one aspect of the patient's total functioning. Table 7.7 shows examples of health problem control outcomes.

Overall health outcomes, on the other hand, indicate at least in part the achievement of providers in terms of total patient health status and functional ability. At this level, specific health problems are considered one factor among many responsible for the patient's level of function. Although this outcome has been most often emphasized in the quality assurance projects reported, it is the most difficult one for physicians to grasp because of the traditional medical orientation toward isolated health problems. Likewise, the complexity of associated factors generally considered outside the range of the responsibility of medical care has discouraged interest in this aspect. However, there is considerable potential for medical practitioners to improve the results of their performance by recognizing the need for increased competence in such skills as patient health education, facilitating patient self-care, and helping patients cope with general problems of lifestyle such as diet, exercise, and stress management.

The basic measure of overall health status used in health accounting is a six level health scale providing a simple and practical means of measuring overall health and disability for a group of patients (see also Chapters 3 and 6). It is applied by means of a questionnaire (see Appendix A), administered by the health accountant in direct patient interviews either in person or by telephone. In some instances, a specially designed version of the questionnaire has also been administered by mail. The patient is asked a series of questions to determine awareness of currently asymptomatic health problems such as high blood pressure or arthritis; recent symptoms or signs related to any physical, emotional, or social problems that have caused discomfort or anxiety or that might indicate present health impairment; inability to perform major life activities more than 25 percent of waking hours, e.g., inability to attend school or to engage in vocational work or retirement activities; and inability to perform activities of daily living more than 25 percent of the time, including dressing, toilet functions, eating, bathing, and ambulation. If the patient has died,

Table 7.7. Examples of health problem control outcomes for quality of care assessment

Health Problem	Followup Period	Measured Outcome[a] (as percent in each category)
Urinary tract infection	6 months	
Recurrence of bacteriuria		37
Recurrence of pyuria		42
Recurrence of symptoms		46
Cholecystectomy	5 years	
Recurrence of original symptoms		
Indigestion		12
Abdominal pain		23
Jaundice		3
Fracture of lower extremity	3 years	
Nonunion (final x-ray)		3
Malunion (final x-ray)		4
Limited motion of ankle or knee		24
Cataractectomy	1 year	
Visual acuity		
20/50 to 20/200		16
< 20/200		2

[a]Problem not adequately controlled.

efforts are made to obtain a copy of the death certificate, to interview the attending physician or a close relative, or to obtain medical chart information related to stated cause of death, circumstances surrounding death, and other relevant factors.

The questionnaire is designed and scored so as to show the highest level of disability that indicates general patient health status as measured by this six level ordinal scale. The aggregate scores for the total sample are arrayed in a frequency distribution to provide an outcome measure for the group as a whole, as shown in the example in Table 7.8.

Outcome Standards. To determine whether measured diagnostic and therapeutic outcomes constitute correctable deficiencies, assessment standards are developed as a benchmark or point of comparison. In principle, standards must be set prior to making assessment measures, so that (1) if agreement regarding standards cannot be reached, the contemplated study can be cancelled, and (2) standards can be obtained without bias from actual findings. These standards then indicate the maximum acceptable level of outcome deficiency; any outcome equal to or better than the standards indicates that further action is not warranted according to the judgment and values of the provider study team (see Chapter 3 for a discussion of standard setting in the light of the evaluation criteria of efficacy, effectiveness, and efficiency of care). If standards are not met, further quality

Table 7.8.   Example of aggregated health status outcomes for a group of cancer of the prostate patients

Health Status	Five year followup Measured Outcome[a] (percent)
Asymptomatic, normal risk	2.3
Asymptomatic, high risk	10.5
Symptomatic	24.4
Restricted	20.9
Dependent	3.5
Dead	38.4

[a]Measured outcomes are always expressed in terms of a percentage distribution over the six level scale.

assurance action is required, whether in the form of additional study to verify assessment results or direct action to improve future outcomes. Like outcome measures, standards are stated in terms of percentages of the diagnostic or therapeutic denominator groups illustrated in Figure 7.1. Table 7.9 shows examples of standards for both diagnostic and therapeutic outcomes.

In the studies reported in Chapters 8–10, most clinic and hospital study teams applied formal or informal group processes in developing their assessment standards (see Chapters 5 and 6 for a discussion of these procedures). Some conducted a thorough literature review on the subject prior to the standard setting session. Most relied primarily upon the knowledge and experience of the team members. A few called in an expert consultant to act as a resource or regular member of the study team.

Diagnostic outcome standards are usually stated as two percentages indicating the maximum acceptable percent of missed diagnoses (false negatives) or misdiagnoses (false positives). Standards for health problem control are usually stated as a single percentage indicating the maximum level of noncontrol that is acceptable, where control is defined in terms of symptom rates, rates of laboratory test results within a given value, or any other measure applicable to the problem status assessed. On the other hand, the overall health status outcome standard is always provided by a frequency distribution of 100 patients over the six level health scale so as to indicate the maximum acceptable disability for the total group; consequently, these standards must not be interpreted to indicate an acceptable percentage at any one level as isolated from the total scale but should be viewed as a whole.

Analysis of Assessment Results

Sampling and Response Rates. The sampling plans describing the group of patients to be identified for outcome assessment in Chapters 8–10 were not in all cases identical to the groups actually identified and observed. However, overall completion rates were generally acceptable, as shown in Tables 7.3 and 7.4. In a few studies, the study population and the population at risk were described or could be inferred but were not enumerated. This also applies to some of the study samples, although these could be approximated from the specific diagnostic and therapeutic denominator groups. Lack of mention of the size of the true negative group was the most frequent omission, especially in earlier studies.

Figure 7.2 indicates the relationship of different denominator

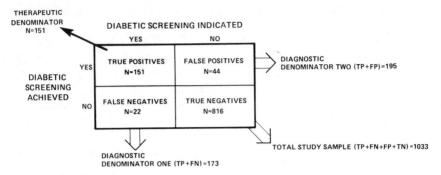

Figure 7.2. Illustration of diagnostic screening outcomes, where diabetic screening was indicated for all true positives and false negatives and achieved for all true positives and false positives.

totals. The response or completion rates achieved indicate the percentage of the planned denominator group for which outcome data were eventually obtained. These rates varied widely across the studies. In the earlier projects, little effort was made to measure or to improve response, but sufficient information was usually available to make a reasonable approximation. The frequent claim to have achieved a 100 percent response or completion rate was not verifiable in a few instances, as indicated on the respective tables in Chapters 8-10. It should be pointed out, though, that subsequent studies have stressed procedures for measuring, documenting, and improving response and completion rates in order to increase the generalizability of the findings.

Computation of completion rates was based on the following formula:

Percent Response

$$= \frac{\text{Actual population for which complete data were obtained}}{\text{Planned population for which data were sought}} (100)$$

The diagnostic and therapeutic denominator groups shown in Chapters 8-10 thus indicate the actual population for which data were obtained. The diagnostic and therapeutic denominator groups underlying false positive and false negative rates, on the other hand, were denominators for the outcome measure percentages actually reported and thus have no direct numerical relationship to the completion rate denominators. Diagnostic and therapeutic completion rates are reported separately, since they represent independent assessment

Table 7.9. Examples of assessment standards for diagnostic and therapeutic outcomes

		Therapeutic Outcome Standards			
Diagnostic Outcome Standards (as percent in each category)	MAS[a]	*Health problem control*[b] (as percent in each category)	MAS[a]	*Health status*[b] (as percent at each level)	MAS[a]
False negatives (diabetes mellitus suspects not screened despite positive screening indications)	5	Fasting blood sugar > 130 mg % average trimonthly assays	20	Asymptomatic, normal risk	15
				Asymptomatic, high risk	25
		Diabetic acidosis during the year	5	Symptomatic	30
				Restricted	17
False positives (diabetes mellitus suspects screened without positive screening indications)	15	Insulin shock during the year	5	Dependent	8
				Dead	5

[a]Maximum acceptable standard.
[b]One year followup of total patient group.

studies and were sometimes derived by independent sampling procedures.

Outcome Analysis. In Chapters 8-10, the results of the health accounting projects are reported in terms of the outcomes observed, the maximum acceptable standards for these outcomes, and the statistical significance of their difference, both observed results and standards being expressed as percents of the given denominator.

Statistical procedures known as goodness of fit tests were used to analyze all differences between observed outcomes and maximum acceptable standards. Goodness of fit tests (one sided) were chosen because it was necessary to compare a sample distribution or proportion (observed outcome) with a theoretical distribution or proportion (maximum acceptable standard).

For diagnostic outcomes, i.e., false positive and false negative rates, and for those therapeutic outcomes stated as health problem control rates, the respective observed rates were compared with the associated maximum acceptable standard using the binomial goodness of fit test (Conover, 1972; Horn, 1977). For therapeutic outcomes measured by the six level health status scale, the observed distribution of patients over that scale was compared with the theoretical distribution postulated by the maximum acceptable standard. Here, the discrete Kolmogorov-Smirnov goodness of fit test (Conover, 1972) was used so as to obtain one level of significance for six discrete pairs of values. These goodness of fit tests were considered the most powerful and appropriate tests available for a comparison of observed outcomes with the maximum acceptable standard (Horn, 1977; Pettitt and Stephens, 1977).

In many of the assessment studies, special findings in addition to overall diagnostic and therapeutic outcome evaluations were reported, e.g., those resulting from classification of the study sample into prognostic risk groups that were observed by individual measures and compared to respective standards. Another aspect reported in several studies was patient satisfaction outcomes.

Summary provider and patient descriptions delineate both the care setting and population characteristics, the former including facility type, location, practice specialty, and financing mechanisms, and the latter demographic descriptors (e.g., age, sex, general socioeconomic characteristics, and enrollee status in prepaid medical plans). Health problem focus is described in terms of overall generic categories, qualified by type, stage, and treatment status as applicable; assessment focus is outlined in terms of diagnostic (or case finding) and therapeutic outcomes, the latter including health problem outcomes in terms of specific symptoms or organ functions and overall patient health status.

SUMMARY

The 56 health accounting projects reported were independently planned and implemented by local physicians and staff, following general guidelines developed by the author and his health accounting team. Their main value lies in demonstrating that outcome assessment studies can be formulated and carried out by practitioners with relatively limited research or evaluation training and that important substantive results and methodological findings can be obtained in primary care clinics and associated hospitals across the nation. Both procedures and results are shown in standard tables to facilitate comparison.

Many of the topics selected for study in the early phases of the health accounting project were determined by informal judgmental processes, usually by the quality assurance coordinator or a small group of interested physicians. It was later established that practicality of care assessment was a major factor in this process. Several clinics also stated that, at first, they preferred to avoid studies where serious deficiencies might be found that would make their group "look bad." As a consequence, early topics often reflected a narrow focus on outcomes of laboratory test utilization, surgical procedures, and specific organic diseases such as anemia, urinary tract infection, and diabetes mellitus, since it seemed that such topics would not involve identification of serious problems of physician management. Despite this handicap, important deficiencies were established, relating to such problems as poor patient compliance and inadequate patient health education. Later, more formal methods for identifying topics and establishing priorities were developed, leading to the selection of topics with greater likelihood of substantial health impact. In subsequent studies not reported here, the predictive validity and reliability of the judgment of providers in selecting high priority topics was documented in 18 projects involving 54 assessment studies (Williamson et al., 1977).

REFERENCES

Clute, K.F. 1963. *The General Practitioner—A Study of Medical Education and Practice in Ontario and Nova Scotia.* Toronto: University of Toronto Press.

Conover, W.J. 1972. A Kolmogorov goodness-of-fit test for discontinuous distributions. *J Am Stat Assoc* 67:591-96.

Densen, P.M. 1972. *Guidelines for Producing Uniform Data for Health Care Plans.* Rockville, Md.: Department of Health, Education and Welfare, Publication No. (HSM) 73-3005.

Horn, S.D. 1977. Goodness-of-fit tests for discrete data—a review and an application to a health impairment scale. *Biometrics* 33:237-48.

Payne, B.C.; Lyons, T.F.; Dwarshins, L.; Kolton, M.; and Morris, W. 1976. *Quality of Medical Care: Evaluation and Improvement.* Health Services Monograph Series T40. Chicago: Hospital Research and Education Trust.

Peterson, O.L.; Andrews, L.P.; Spain, R.S.; and Greenberg, B.G. 1956. An analytic study of North Carolina general practice—1953-1954. *J Med Educ* 31 (12) pt. 2.

Pettitt, A.M., and Stephens, M.A. 1977. The Kolmogorov-Smirnov goodness-of-fit statistic with discrete and grouped data. *Technometrics* 19:205-10.

Williamson, J.W.; Horn, S.D.; Choi, T.; and White, P.E. 1977. Evaluating an outcome-based quality assurance system. Final Project Report, Grant HS01590, National Center for Health Services Research, Department of Health, Education and Welfare. Baltimore: The Johns Hopkins School of Hygiene and Public Health (processed).

Chapter 8

Health Accounting Outcome Studies: Organic Disease and Fractures

In this chapter the results of 35 health accounting projects relating to organic medical disease and fractures are presented. Here, the categories most frequently chosen by the participating clinics were the stress-related problems of hypertension and peptic ulcer (11 projects incorporating 20 assessment studies), followed by infectious diseases (10 projects, 18 studies), and neoplastic, endocrine, and cerebro-cardiovascular diseases (4 projects each for a total of 16 studies). Fractures were studied in two projects. Assessment focus was variously on the outcomes of diagnostic or therapeutic management or both. (See Chapter 7 for a discussion of outcome categories.)

STRESS RELATED PROBLEMS

Topics involving problems related to lifestyle and self-imposed risks have attracted widespread attention in recent years. Hypertension thus was a frequently studied topic. It is also possible, however, that the seeming practicality of studying hypertension was as much of a factor as its theoretical interest and medical importance, since only one other topic (peptic ulcer) was selected in the general category of diseases presumably related to stress.

Hypertension
Topic. Elevated blood pressure was the most frequent health problem studied, with a total of ten projects implemented by a group of twelve clinics. This choice was probably due to the widespread

acceptance of the efficacy of treatment, to the seriousness of complications, to high prevalence, to increasing evidence of its neglect in medical practice, and to the apparent simplicity of identifying patients with this problem. Hypertension was variously defined, but all projects included patients who either had elevated blood pressure readings (recorded in charts or taken prospectively) or normal readings but a history of diagnosed and/or treated hypertension.

The providers in these studies were mainly primary care physicians in four fee for service and eight prepaid clinics, and including the staff of one city hospital emergency room. In two instances, two small adjacent clinics pooled their patients for purposes of the study. Of ten completed projects, four related to poverty populations and six to working and/or middle class populations. All patients were adults, both male and female, generally between ages 35 and 65.

In eight assessment studies, the focus was on outcomes of the diagnostic process in terms of assessing missed diagnoses (false negatives) only; two studies assessed misdiagnoses (false positives) as well. False negatives were defined as patients requiring but not receiving adequate blood pressure management, i.e., those whose blood pressure was out of control, either due to absence of any treatment or due to inadequate treatment currently provided. False positives were defined as patients receiving but not requiring management, i.e., those erroneously labeled as having hypertension. Most clinics elected not to study false positives, since this would have involved stopping medication for extended periods.

Therapeutic outcome assessment was confined to the overall health status of the patient groups studied. This measure, made uniformly in nine studies, provides crude but interesting comparative data. In addition, educational outcomes were examined in two studies in terms of patient and physician knowledge, behavior, and attitudes.

Design. In seven studies, the design involved a retrospective chart review to identify all patients at risk (usually defined only by age, e.g., 35 to 65 years) within a specified time interval or up to a specified sample size. Three studies were prospective, focusing on consecutive adult walk-in patients at risk who were subsequently screened for hypertension. In these three studies, new or untreated suspects were followed to confirm the diagnosis by consecutive readings at spaced intervals.

Diagnostic outcomes were measured by classifying all patients at risk on either or both of two independent lists. The first included all patients at risk requiring management (or altered management) of hypertension. The criteria ranged from simple single readings of diastolic pressure in excess of 90 to 110 mm Hg to elaborate criteria standardized by age, blood pressure cuff width, and three consecutive readings in defined patient postures at specified time intervals.

The second list (usually developed by chart review) included all patients meeting specified criteria and receiving hypertension management, whether or not it was required. Patients appearing on both lists were labeled "true positives," those only on the first list "false negatives," and in one study, those only on the second list "false positives." In the latter study (Study 10), diagnostic outcomes emphasized detection of one complication of hypertension—heart failure—false negatives including hypertensive patients requiring but not receiving heart failure management, and false positives patients being treated for heart failure without adequate justification. One clinic (Study 29) in addition developed a system of weights to assign each hypertensive in the sample to one of three prognostic groups, as shown in Table 8.1.

Therapeutic outcomes for all patients were measured by contacting each personally to measure general health status as a crude index of quality of individual life and function. Using a standard questionnaire, each patient was indexed at one of six levels, ranging from asymptomatic status over increasing levels of disability interfering with the achievement of current life goals to death (for a detailed

Table 8.1. Prognostic weights for hypertensive patients

Study 29			
Factor	*Weights*	*Factor*	*Weights*
Age of onset		*Complications*	
< 20 years	40	Hyperlipidemia	20
20 to 35 years	30	Diabetes mellitus	20
36 to 50 years	20	Renal disease	20
> 50 years	10	Arteriosclerotic heart disease	20
Sex		Arteriosclerosis	20
Male	20	Hypertensive cardio- vascular disease	20
Female	0	Cerebrovascular accident	20
		Peripheral vascular disease	20
Race		Gout	20
Black	20		
White	0		

Best Prognostic Group	0–40 points
Moderate Prognostic Group	41–100 points
Worst Prognostic Group	> 100 points

description of the health and functional ability scale used, see Chapter 6). A health profile of the group was then established in terms of the frequency distribution of patients at the various levels.

Educational outcomes were measured in two clinics by a patient awareness questionnaire unique to each clinic and consisting of a series of questions such as the following:

- Have you ever been informed by a physician that you had high blood pressure?
- If you have hypertension and feel symptom-free, can you still be in serious immediate danger of complications from high blood pressure?

Similar questions related to attitudes and behavior. Aspects of compliance, such as taking pills and keeping appointments, were verified in two studies by pill counts and clinic records.

In all clinics, standards were developed by group consensus of clinic staff serving on the study teams. Clinic teams generally were limited to physicians, though in more recent projects, nurses and clinic administrative personnel were included as well. Standards consisted of maximum acceptable rates for false negatives, false positives, and maximum acceptable total group disability expressed by a hypothetical distribution of 100 patients across the six level health scale.

Results. *Clinical   Outcomes.* Observed   diagnostic   outcomes failed to meet maximum acceptable standards (MAS) in all but two studies, as shown in Table 8.2. The discrepancy between observed results and standards was usually sufficiently large to be apparent even in the absence of tests of significance. It is of interest that the maximum acceptable standards set for the proportion of hypertensive patients requiring but not receiving adequate management ranged from 2 percent to 19 percent, with an average of 7 percent. The two least stringent standards (15 and 19 percent) were set in fee for service clinics; the most stringent standard (2 percent) was set in three prepaid clinics. Measured results ranged from 3 percent false negatives in the emergency room of a midwestern city hospital to 46 percent in a large metropolitan clinic, with an average of 25 percent.

The clinic that weighted hypertensives according to prognosis was one of the two where measured diagnostic outcomes met the established standards (Study 29; Table 8.2). However, among the 40 in the 133 patient sample who were considered to have the poorest prognosis, one in three appeared to receive inadequate care in

Table 8.2.   Health care assessment results in ten studies of hypertension management in adults

Provider Characteristics	Patient and Sample Characteristics	Diagnostic Outcomes[a] (as percent in each category)		Therapeutic Outcomes (as percent at each level)			Sample Size (n) and Completion Rate (percent)			
		Obs	MAS		Obs***	MAS	Diagnostic n	%	Therapeutic n	%
Study 10 Facility 3										
Emergency room of a city hospital affiliated with university school of medicine in an eastern metropolis. 71 house staff	Urban poverty class adults. Retrospective sampling of consecutive walk-ins with BPb > 100; 1 year followup	(n = 98) False negatives 3	5	(n = 87) Asymptomatic, normal and high risk	8	57	100	98	100	87
		(n = 95) False positives 0	5	Symptomatic	44	18				
				Restricted	26	10				
				Dependent	1	3				
				Dead	21	10				
		Obs	MAS		Obs*	MAS				
Study 20 Facility 7										
Private fee for service clinic in suburban eastern town. 20 physicians	Middle and working class adults. Retrospective sampling of new clinic admissions in 6 months with BPb > 100; 6 month followup	(n = 120) False negatives 30***15		(n = 114) Asymptomatic, normal risk	29	33	157	76	137	83
				Asymptomatic, high risk	38	44				
				Symptomatic	23	12				
				Restricted	5	4				
				Dependent	1	3				
				Dead	4	4				

(Continued)

Table 8.2.   continued

Provider Characteristics	Patient and Sample Characteristics	Diagnostic Outcomes[a] (as percent in each category)		Therapeutic Outcomes (as percent at each level)			Sample Size (n) and Completion Rate (percent)			
		Obs	MAS		Obs	MAS	Diagnostic n	%	Therapeutic n	%
Study 23 Facility 8										
Fee for service and prepaid private group practice in a rural eastern town. 197 physicians	Working class adults. Retrospective review of clinic charts for patients with BP^b > 100; 1 year followup			(n = 99)					100	99
				Asymptomatic, normal risk	4	12				
				Asymptomatic, high risk	28	23				
				Symptomatic	39	44				
				Restricted	19	9				
				Dependent	3	6				
				Dead	6	5				
Study 29 Facility 10										
Fee for service and prepaid clinic in a rural midwestern town. 16 physicians	Middle and working class adults. Retrospective chart review for all patients diagnosed as hypertensive in past 6 months with BP^b > 95; 6 month followup	(n = 133) False negatives 16	19	(n = 121)			150	89	133	91
				Asymptomatic, normal and high risk	69.5	23				
				Symptomatic	19	39				
				Restricted	8	23				
				Dependent	1	7				
				Dead	2.5	8				

Study 36 Facility 12

	Obs	MAS		Obs***	MAS	n	%	n	%
Prepaid university affiliated HMO in eastern city. 4 physicians			Poverty class adults. Retrospective chart review for all hypertensive patients seen in 30 month period with BPb > 90; 1 year followup					158	94
			(n = 149)						
			Asymptomatic, normal risk	11	3				
			Asymptomatic, high risk	28	74				
			Symptomatic	40	14				
			Restricted	16	7				
			Dependent	2	2				
			Dead	3	0				

Study 43 Facility 15 and 16

	Obs	MAS		Obs***	MAS	n	%	n	%
Prepaid corporate clinics in western metropolitan area. 17 physicians	41***	2	Middle and working class adults. Prospective sampling of all walk-in patients with diagnoses of BPb > 100; 6 month followup of subsample. False negatives			570	100	100	83
			(n = 83)						
			Asymptomatic, normal risk	3	22				
			Asymptomatic, high risk	10	30				
			Symptomatic	60	13				
			Restricted	19	27				
			Dependent	8	7				
			Dead	0	1				

Study 46 Facility 17

	Obs	MAS		Obs**	MAS	n	%	n	%
Prepaid corporate clinic in western metropolitan region. 17 physicians	42***	2	Poverty class adults. Retrospective chart review of all patients seen in 11 months for diagnoses of BPb > 110; 6 month followup of subsample. False negatives			860	100	163	67
			(n = 109)						
			Asymptomatic, normal risk	2	0				
			Asymptomatic, high risk	16	31				
			Symptomatic	61	50				
			Restricted	21	13				
			Dependent	0	3				
			Dead	0	3				

(Continued)

Table 8.2.   continued

Provider Characteristics	Patient and Sample Characteristics	Diagnostic Outcomes[a] (as percent in each category)		Therapeutic Outcomes (as percent at each level)			Sample Size (n) and Completion Rate (percent)			
							Diagnostic		Therapeutic	
		Obs	MAS		Obs***	MAS	n	%	n	%
Study 47 Facility 18										
Prepaid corporate clinic in western metropolitan region. 5 physicians	Poverty class adults. Prospective sample of all walk-in patients seen in 2 months for diagnoses of $BP_D > 110$; 2 month followup of 202 patients	(n = 215) False negatives 46***	5	(n = 100)			725	100	202	50
				Asymptomatic, normal risk	5	10				
				Asymptomatic, high risk	6	21				
				Symptomatic	32	50				
				Restricted	49	13				
				Dependent	7	3				
				Dead	1	3				
Study 50 Facility 19 and 20										
Prepaid corporate clinics in western metropolitan region. 21 physicians	Working class adults. Prospective sampling of all walk-in patients seen in 1 month period for diagnoses of $BP_D > 110$	(n = 103) False negatives 31***	2	(n = 83)			324	100	103	81
				Asymptomatic, normal risk	0	0				
				Asymptomatic, high risk	37	84				
				Symptomatic	48	12				
				Restricted	11	2				
				Dependent	4	1				
				Dead	0	1				

Study 55 Facility 22		Obs	MAS		
			n	%	n	%
Prepaid university HMO in eastern metropolitan region. 17 physicians	Poverty class adults. Retrospective sampling of charts for enrollees seen at clinic for diagnoses of BP^b > 100	False negatives (n = 178)	19***	6	297	100
		False positives (n = 154)	6	4		

^{a}False negatives are defined as patients requiring but not receiving adequate blood pressure management, except in Study 10, which included management of heart failure among hypertensive patients; false positives are defined as patients receiving but not requiring blood pressure management.

^{b}BP = Diastolic blood pressure.

Note: In Tables 8.2–8.21, the abbreviations Obs and MAS denote, respectively, observed results and maximum acceptable standards. See Chapter 7 for methods used to determine statistical significance.

*P < 0.05
**P < 0.01
***P < 0.001

Table 8.3. Diagnostic and therapeutic outcomes for hypertensive patients by prognostic group

	Study 29							
	Diagnostic Outcomes[a] (as percent false negatives)	Therapeutic Outcomes[b] (as percent at each level of the six level health scale)						
Prognostic Group		1	2	3	4	5	6
Best	(n = 45)	(n = 38)						
	Observed	11		92		5	3	0
	MAS	15		84		10	2	4
Moderate	(n = 48)	(n = 45)						
	Observed	8		94		4	0	2
	MAS	20		68		20	4	8
Worst	(n = 40)	(n = 38)						
	Observed	30		79		16	0	5
	MAS	20		34		40	14	12

[a]Diastolic blood pressure > 100mm Hg (management required but not being achieved).
[b]Six month followup.

relation to blood pressure control (see Table 8.3), whereas the maximum acceptable standard would allow only one in five to be thus neglected.

Overall health disability exceeded maximum impairment standards in seven out of ten studies. Aggregating all clinics except one (Facility 10, where the team either did not understand or did not take seriously the standard setting task), nearly 25 percent of the hypertensive patients sampled were unable to perform their major life activity on followup, one out of five of those who were disabled having died. This measured finding was significantly worse than the MAS average of 16 percent.

Behavioral Outcomes. Tables 8.4 and 8.5 present aggregated educational results as measured and observed in two clinics. The findings in Table 8.4 provide rather clear presumptive evidence for the measured deficiencies in terms of health outcomes. With regard to the patients, the proportion not understanding the fact that danger of death or complications of hypertension are not necessarily related to symptoms (a question not asked in Study 29, however) is closely associated with low compliance in taking antihypertensive medication. Poor patient understanding of these facts is most likely responsible for the inadequate blood pressure control rates in these

Table 8.4. Questionnaire results for patient knowledge and behavior regarding hypertension

Knowledge Items	Study 29 (n = 110)	Studies 43 and 50 (n = 148[a])
Unaware that they had hypertension	—	16
Unaware that treatment works (is efficacious)	6	—
Unaware that hypertension is a serious risk to health	6	9
Unaware of the form or dosage of the drug they were receiving to control hypertension	7	20
Unaware of the possible toxic effects of the drug they were receiving to control hypertension	—	81
Unaware that the danger of hypertension is not related only to symptoms	—	93
Total number of patients with inadequate information[b]	7	95

Behavior Items	Study 29 (n = 110)	Studies 43 and 50 (n = 148[a])
Not keeping regular appointments	64	—
Not taking any medication for hypertension	16	39
Taking medication for hypertension sporadically	8	25
Taking medication for hypertension only if symptoms occur	—	16
Total number taking inadequate medication[b]	24	80

[a] Extrapolated.
[b] Counting each patient once.
— Not asked.

Table 8.5. Questionnaire results on physician knowledge and attitudes regarding hypertension

		Studies 43 and 50	
Knowledge Items	*Physicians (n = 14)*	*Attitude Items*	*Physicians (n = 14)*
Inadequate drug information	0	Omitted the education of patients on aspects of ideal care for hypertension	11
Unaware that danger of hypertension is not related to symptoms	4	Questioned the criteria for hypertension determined in a study by the Veterans Administration	5
Overestimated national control of hypertension and compliance	8		
Overestimated control of hypertension or compliance by own patients	10	Rejected clinical diagnostic standards for evaluating the outcome of treatment	1
Total with inadequate information[a]	11	Total who were possibly deficient[a]	11

[a]Counting each physician once.

studies. With regard to physicians (Table 8.5), it was evident that while having adequate clinical knowledge (such as tested in licensure or certification examinations), they did not seem to be aware of equally important facts regarding the poor compliance of their own patients or the importance of health education in managing hypertension.

Implications. The clinical implications of these ten studies in twelve institutions seem serious. In spite of the crude measures obtained by clinical personnel and health accountants, there is little doubt that the maximum acceptable standards for diagnostic and therapeutic outcomes were not met in all but two instances, and in one of these, standards were seriously exceeded in relation to a subset of 40 patients judged at high risk and having evidence of complications. It seems clear that subsequent definitive study was indicated in each of the projects in order to identify correctable determinants of deficient outcomes. However, only four clinics conducted a followup and identified specific factors likely to be responsible for deficient outcomes; if corrected, these factors might have proved both necessary and sufficient for obtaining adequate blood pressure control and related reduction in mortality and complication rates. The patient and physician educational outcomes assessed in two clinics represent a first step in this direction. Here, too, the findings strongly indicate inadequate compliance and seriously deficient understanding on the part of both physicians and patients.

Health outcomes in terms of overall disability were more serious than anticipated, despite the fact that the average followup interval was only six months to one year and that the risk of complications in this condition can extend over many years. That immediate investigation of overall health determinants was indicated seemed obvious, but this was usually not achieved. The lack of motivation to pursue this deficiency would itself seem to require serious followup investigation.

The quality assurance implications of the study of this health problem are equally significant. Many professional groups elect to study outcomes of hypertension management without realizing many of the hidden complexities of this topic. The most serious problem involves measurement of representative blood pressure levels. Three isolated blood pressure readings, however accurate, may not be representative of the mean pressure experienced by the patient throughout the year. Yet the validity of conclusions regarding blood pressure control drawn from a limited sample of readings may well depend upon such considerations. Aside from the problems regarding the number and timing of blood pressure readings, the precise conditions at any one reading are usually not reported. Was the patient sitting up or lying down? What prior rest period was achieved? What size blood pressure cuff was used? Finally, which pressure levels are to be considered abnormal is a subject of contention. If diastolic readings in excess of 115 mm Hg are applied, few will argue about false positives, but the number of false negatives may be serious. Yet setting the cutting level at 90 mm Hg, while eliminating most false negatives, will include many more false positives. Such problems make hypertension measurement, diagnoses, and control much more complicated than is usually recognized.

On the other hand, that a variety of quality assurance teams in a wide range of multispecialty clinics were able to apply health accounting methods after a minimum of training and guidance and could obtain generally similar results confirming the magnitude and seriousness of identified outcome deficiencies seems to confirm the feasibility of the study methods. In most of the twelve clinics improvement action seemed indicated, confirming the tentative validity both of standards and of assessment measures. Also, these results provided evidence supporting the outcome assessment approach as a method of identifying areas of potential health improvement, at least insofar as hypertensive patients are concerned.

Peptic Ulcer

Topic. The second stress related disease studied in the first phase of the health accounting projects, peptic ulcer, was chosen by one clinic serving an urban industrial population in the Midwest. The providers were physicians on the staff of a fee for service multi-specialty group clinic. The patients studied were middle class (60 percent) and working class (40 percent), mostly male (70 percent), and with few exceptions between age 30 and 69 (average, late 40s). The focus of this study was on outcomes of therapeutic manage-ment, and the study team elected assessment of patients having had an episode of peptic ulcer as confirmed by a positive x-ray report.

Design. Sampling in Study 18 was based on radiology report files, and diagnoses of initial peptic ulcer episodes were confirmed by chart review. One hundred consecutive patients seen three to five years prior to the study were to be contacted and interviewed. The patients actually followed were divided into two prognostic groups based on followup findings related to six factors (stress, alcohol/cigarette use, compliance, complications, other major disease, and x-ray followup). The best prognostic group (acute nonrecurrent) consisted of 48 patients, and the worst prognostic group (chronic recurrent) of 26 patients. A patient satisfaction questionnaire was applied to all patients studied.

Overall health outcomes were measured by assigning each patient to one of the six levels of the health and functional ability scale, and the frequency distribution of patients across this scale was com-pared to the maximum acceptable standard (MAS) developed by clinic staff on the study team. It should be pointed out that as in most other studies discussed here, this standard, representing the maximum group impairment that the staff would accept without electing to make a more detailed inquiry into this problem area, does not represent the health outcomes the staff expected to find; instead, it provided an indication of their values regarding the level of group impairment beyond which further assessment effort on their part would be warranted.

Results. The comparison of measured group findings to maximum acceptable standards revealed serious discrepancies, with 5 percent unexpected deaths and only 66 percent of patients asymptomatic, as compared to an acceptable minimum of 83 percent, as shown in Table 8.6. The surprising finding was that all the deaths were among the 48 acute patients who supposedly had the best prognosis (Table 8.7). Questions were raised as to whether death had in fact been related to the ulcer in three of the four patients who died. The reported results of the questionnaire on patient satisfaction revealed that 70 percent of patients indicated they were satisfied with the care provided.

Implications. From a clinical point of view, far more disability was found in this study than was considered acceptable by the clinic staff's own standards, and the fact that the better prognostic group produced all of the deaths raises questions as to the validity of the prognostic factors specified and measured. Also, in view of the preponderance of middle-aged patients who should have been active in their vocational pursuits, a more focused inquiry into the causes of what was clearly a deficient outcome would have appeared crucial.

The quality assurance implications of this study were disheartening. Staff involvement was especially poor. Only one member of the original study team was present when the results were reported to the clinic staff. Repeated efforts to continue to identify correctable determinants of the unacceptably high symptom, bedridden, and mortality outcomes failed, although the often observed initial skepticism regarding the process of formulating health outcome standards had not been much greater than in other clinics. Due to lack of involvement and failure to follow up on assessment findings in this study, as well as unsatisfactory participation in two other studies, this clinic decided not to continue the health accounting program.

INFECTIOUS DISEASE

Infectious disease provides an assessment topic of particular interest because of the potential for identifying a specific etiological agent and the availability of definitive treatment interventions such as antibiotics. Among the projects conducted in the first ten years of health accounting, 10 focused on this topic, encompassing a total of 18 assessment studies.

Table 8.6.   Health care assessment results in a study of peptic ulcers in adults

Provider Characteristics	Patient and Sample Characteristics	Therapeutic Outcomes (as percent at each level)		Sample Size (n) and Completion Rate (percent)	
			Obs*** MAS	n	%
Study 18 Facility 6					
Fee for service clinic in mid-western city. 26 physicians	Middle and working class adults, mainly 30–69 years. Retrospective sampling of radiology file and charts for consecutive peptic ulcer diagnoses; 3–5 year followup	(n = 74) Asymptomatic, normal and high risk	66 83	100	74
		Symptomatic	23 11		
		Restricted	3 5		
		Dependent	3 0		
		Dead	5 0		

***P < 0.001

Table 8.7. Therapeutic outcomes for peptic ulcer patients by prognostic group

	Study 18			
	Best Prognostic Group[a] (n = 48)		Worst Prognostic Group[b] (n = 26)	
Therapeutic Outcomes (as percent at each level)	Observed	MAS	Observed	MAS
Asymptomatic, normal and high risk	79	97	42	57
Symptomatic	13	3	42	27
Restricted	0	0	8	15
Dependent	0	0	8	0.5
Dead	8	0	0	0.5

[a]Initial diagnosed episode of acute peptic ulcer.
[b]Previous or recurrent diagnosed episodes of peptic ulcer.

Urinary Tract Infections

Topic. The health problem selected for six projects was urinary tract infection. The facilities were private fee for service clinics under varying auspices and one university medical center, in locations ranging from a south central town to a western metropolis. Clinics and their associated hospitals were included in three of the projects. The patient populations varied from consecutive walk-in patients to obstetrical inpatients at time of delivery. Average patient age was in the 30s, with an overall balance between poverty, working, and middle socioeconomic classes.

Patients were predominantly female, though one clinic stressed males over 60 years of age. The focus of study was on the outcomes of diagnostic management (5 studies) and on the health outcomes of therapeutic management (4 studies). Missed diagnoses (false negatives) were studied in five and misdiagnoses (false positives) in four instances. One study was not carried through beyond the initial stages (Study 37).

Design. Sampling was based on prospective study of all clinic walk-ins or hospital admissions in Studies 7, 8, 30, and 49 and on retrospective study of hospital patients in Study 40. Diagnostic management outcomes were usually determined by comparing independent history and laboratory tests results with recorded or implied diagnoses in the patient's medical chart.

Urinary tract infections were defined as bacteriuria established by quantitative urine cultures in all five studies, but were restricted to symptomatic patients in one study. In all studies, two independent urine specimens were obtained and tested, the first usually by screening smears, testuria assay, or culture and the second (if the first test was positive) by quantitative culture. The attending physician's diagnosis was obtained from chart review. The followup interval ranged from six weeks postpartum in the retrospective study to six months posthospital admission in one of the prospective studies, with an average interval of two and a half months.

Therapeutic management outcomes related to overall health status were determined by independent interview of the patient in three studies. Health problem outcomes were determined by repeat urine cultures in one study. Assessment standards were established by consensual clinic or hospital staff team agreement in terms of the maximum acceptable percentage of false negatives and false positives for diagnostic outcomes and of the hypothetical distribution of 100 patients over the health scale to represent the highest level of group disability that would be tolerated without recommending more detailed subsequent study.

Results. Diagnostic outcome assessment revealed universal deficiencies in terms of missed diagnoses (false negatives); these ranged from 34 to 83 percent (average 55 percent) above the maximum acceptable limits (0 to 15 percent, with an average of 8 percent), as shown in Table 8.8. Deficiencies in terms of misdiagnoses (false positives) were noted in two of four clinics.

Therapeutic outcomes were considered deficient in two of the four studies. The major problem related to bacteriuria in Study 30 and to recurrent symptoms in Study 7. In Study 40, it was found that of 24 patients hospitalized for complications prior to onset of labor, in 12 cases this was due to urinary tract infections. Analysis by the clinic staff indicated that most of these symptomatic exacerbations were preventable, since these patients had clearly been inadequately treated if they had been treated at all. On the other hand, overall health outcomes in Study 40 (as shown in Table 8.8) did not exceed maximum acceptable impairment standards.

Implications. Diagnostic management was seriously inadequate in all clinics studied as judged by the staff physicians' own standards. These findings have been reported frequently in the literature and are difficult to explain. It is possible that while physicians will state that such urinary tract infections are serious and that treatment produces significant health benefit, they nonetheless doubt the efficacy of

Table 8.8.   Health care assessment results in five studies of urinary tract infections in adults

Provider Characteristics	Patient and Sample Characteristics	Diagnostic Outcomes[a] (as percent in each category)		Therapeutic Outcomes (as percent at each level)	Sample Size (n) and Completion Rate (percent)			
					Diagnostic		Therapeutic	
		Obs	MAS		n	%	n	%
Study 7 Facility 1								
Fee for service clinic and hospital in midwestern city. 114 physicians	Middle and working class adults. Prospective sampling of hospital admissions (6 months); 6 month followup for subsample with positive test results	(n = 265) False negatives 71*** (n = 110) False positives 29**	15 20	(n = 33)[b] Treated and cured 39 Not treated and cured 24 Treated and not cured 21 Not treated and not cured 15	268	99	—	—
Study 8 Facility 2		Obs	MAS		n	%	n	%
University medical center in midwestern metropolis. 698 physicians	Poverty class adults. Prospective sampling of consecutive new clinic admissions; 3 month post-admission follow-up	(n = 18) False negatives 56*** (n = 8) False positives 0	15 20		150	89		

(Continued)

Table 8.8.   continued

Provider Characteristics	Patient and Sample Characteristics	Diagnostic Outcomes[a] (as percent in each category)		Therapeutic Outcomes (as percent at each level)			Sample Size (n) and Completion Rate (percent)			
							Diagnostic		Therapeutic	
		Obs	MAS		Obs***	MAS	n	%	n	%
Study 30 Facility 10										
Private fee for service clinic in a midwestern town. 16 physicians	Middle and working class adults. Prospective sampling of consecutive walk-ins with acute cystitis; 1 month post-visit followup	(n = 28) False negatives 47*** (n = 53) False positives 30***	0 0	(n = 100) Asymptomatic, normal and high risk Symptomatic Restricted Dependent Dead	72 28 0 0 0	100 0 0 0 0	144	100	144	69
Study 40 Facility 13		Obs	MAS		Obs	MAS	n	%	n	%
Private fee for service clinic in south central rural town. 50 physicians	Working class adult females. Retrospective review of laboratory test reports for 150 deliveries with positive testuria assays confirmed by culture; 6 weeks postpartum followup	(n = 124) False negatives 34***	0	(n = 124) Asymptomatic, normal and high risk Symptomatic Restricted Dependent Dead	60 23 15 2 0	62 25 10 3 0	150	83	150	83

	Obs	MAS		Obs	MAS		n	%	n	%	n	%
Study 49 Facility 19 and 20												
Corporate fee for service clinic in western metropolis. 21 physicians. Working class patients. Prospective sample of consecutive walk-in females (> age 8) and males (> age 60) screened by urine cultures; 1 month postvisit follow-up									502	34	127	100
(n = 127) False negatives	83***	5										
(n = 21) False positives	0	17										
(n = 127) Asymptomatic, normal risk				38	28							
Asymptomatic, high risk				23	20							
Symptomatic				28	20							
Restricted				10	22							
Dependent				1	8							
Dead				0	2							
Study 37ᶜ Facility 12												
Prepaid university HMO in large eastern city. 4 physicians. Poverty class adults. Prospective sampling of consecutive walk-ins having urinary tract infections in a 1 year period; (1–2 year followup planned)												

[a] Diagnostic screening outcomes, where false negatives refer to absence of diagnosis or treatment of urinary tract infection despite positive screening culture and false positives to diagnosis and/or treatment despite negative screening culture.

[b] Health problem outcomes; health scale not applied. Cured cases determined by three negative independent urine cultures or smears taken > 1 week apart.

[c] Study 37 was not completed.

— Size of subsample not stated.

**P < 0.01
***P < 0.001

treating this common condition. A recent review by Dershewitz (1975) confirms the present controversy regarding efficacy. There is little hard evidence that treatment of asymptomatic bacteriuria prolongs life or prevents chronic pyelonephritis and renal failure. On the other hand, it is probably safe to state that treatment of bacteriuria can prevent symptomatic episodes of urinary tract infection and perhaps hospitalization for acute or exacerbated pyelonephritis. Study 40 seemed to support this contention at least in regard to urinary tract infection in pregnancy. The physicians conducting the studies reported here apparently did judge available treatment modes to be sufficiently efficacious to warrant detection and management of this condition.

The equivocal therapeutic outcome results in this group of studies can probably be explained by the small number of studies reported here and by the relatively short followup interval (4 to 6 weeks) in the two studies indicating no significant discrepancies between results and standards. The health standards did seem inordinately low in one of the latter instances (Study 49) and may have been invalid. The team standard indicated that they would not be concerned if as much as 30 percent of a group of patients with urinary tract infection were sufficiently disabled as to be out of work one month after their clinic visit followup. In the second instance, the standard seemed inordinately high, indicating little judgmental input. This clinic (Study 30) implied that anything short of complete cure of all urinary tract infections would warrant further study.

On the other hand, these assessment studies of outcomes of clinical management of urinary tract infections were surprisingly good for an initial effort. The findings were probably valid, and improvement implications were clear. However, lack of sophistication was indicated by the absence of any literature support regarding treatment efficacy and the difficulties in sampling in most of the clinics. Sample frames were defined loosely, and response rates were mixed; a wider sampling base, especially one including total enrolled groups, might produce better results. Further, a standardization of diagnostic screening procedures seemed to be indicated. The sensitivity and specificity of screening tests required better documentation (Medical Letter, 1974), especially for the combinations of diagnostic tests and methods illustrated in this series of studies.

The most unsatisfactory aspect was the lack of physician interest in an exploration of correctable determinants of the outcome deficiencies measured, which was offset in only one instance (Study 7), where the clinic studied determinants of the deficiency and attempted improvement to bring diagnostic outcomes within standards.

If urinary tract infections are worth diagnosing, a 55 percent average rate of missed diagnoses seems serious. The fact that in only one case was any further inquiry conducted or an effort made to effect improvement indicates an apathy that could threaten any quality assurance approach.

In the specific facility where subsequent action was taken, a two year effort failed to significantly improve individual physician performance. As a result, the staff voted to delegate authority to screen and confirm the diagnosis of bacteriuria to laboratory personnel. All hospital admissions were to be thus screened, using stained uncentrifuged urine smears and followup quantitative cultures for all positive smear results, and the physician was to be informed of confirmed infections. While this may solve the problem of detection and missed diagnoses, the question of improved therapeutic management remains to be studied.

Bacterial Pneumonia in Children

Topic. Bacterial pneumonia was the health problem selected in one clinic, a university administered health maintenance organization in a newly developed town adjacent to an eastern metropolis. The patient population consisted of children seen in the pediatric clinic and treated for bacterial pneumonia. They averaged 3.9 years, with 15 aged less than 1 year; 42 were male and 48 female, all of middle class background. The study focused on outcomes of therapeutic management. The topic had been chosen because of its frequency, importance, and the established efficacy of treatment in altering the course of the illness.

Design. Prospective sampling of one hundred consecutive pediatric clinic visits in an eight month period by patients having a diagnosis of bacterial pneumonia and receiving antibiotic treatment provided the study group. Health outcomes were measured at a two month followup interval by administration of a questionnaire to the mothers of the children sampled. Each patient was categorized at one of the six levels of the standard health scale developed in the health accounting project (see Chapter 6). Outcome standards were established by group judgment in terms of a distribution of 100 patients over the health scale, indicating the maximum acceptable group disability at two months after diagnosis and treatment.

Results. Measured health outcomes were significantly worse than maximum acceptable standards, as shown in Table 8.9. Subsequent analysis indicated that continued coughing was the major aspect of this deficient outcome. A followup study of these children by repeat x-rays and clinical examination revealed no serious pathology that warranted further medical management, and it was concluded that the original outcome standards had been too stringent and should be altered for future assessment.

As part of the original outcome study, the patients had been classi-fied into three prognostic groups in order of increasing seriousness. Prognostic determinants included presence of asthma or other major chest disease, cystic fibrosis, sickle cell disease, immunodeficiency, whether the patient had been seen in the clinic before, and "other minor predisposing factors." The total group showed 58 in the best prognostic group (no negative factors); 41 were in the intermediate group (asthma, not being seen before, or other minor factors), and 1 was in the worst group (major chest disease). Measured health out-comes were indeed worse in the latter two groups. An ancillary find-ing that one in five patients had not received a followup check was felt to be a serious deficiency.

Implications. The medical management of the group of children studied proved excellent in that no correctable determinants of defi-cient outcomes were found. Even the 21 cases not receiving a fol-lowup check revealed that no further action was necessary when they were brought in for further study.

Quality assurance implications of this study are more meaningful. Childhood pneumonia is a difficult topic to assess due to the fact that bacterial etiology often cannot be differentiated from viral etiol-ogy except by blood cultures or endotracheal aspiration. Throat cul-tures are notoriously misleading, both in terms of false negatives and false positives. If most such patients have viral disease, the potential benefits of physician management may be rather limited. Further, there was serious reason, in this project, to question the judgment of the clinic staff in selecting this topic as one that might provide sig-nificant improvement. More than one team member later admitted to not having taken the judgment process quite seriously and to having deliberately picked a topic where the pediatrics staff would probably look good.

Also, this study is an illustration of inappropriate health outcome standards. The staff was genuinely surprised to discover that the resolution of pneumonia in children can take up to four months in terms of symptoms, especially coughing. It was agreed that if the present standards were to be applied at a four month followup inter-val, as opposed to the two month interval used in this study, a

Table 8.9.   Health care assessment results in a study of bacterial pneumonia in children

Provider Characteristics	Patient and Sample Characteristics	Therapeutic Outcomes (as percent at each level)		Sample Size (n) and Completion Rate (percent)	
		Obs **	MAS	n	%
Study 15 Facility 5					
Prepaid university HMO in an eastern town in metropolitan region. 45 physicians	Middle class children. Prospective sampling (8 months) of consecutive pediatric clinic walk-in patients diagnosed as having bacterial pneumonia; 2 month followup	(n = 100) Asymptomatic, normal and		100[a]	100
		high risk 80	96		
		Symptomatic 19	3.5		
		Restricted 0	0		
		Dependent 1	0		
		Dead 0	0.5		

[a]Ninety-five children, of whom five contracted bacterial pneumonia twice.

**P < 0.01

finding of over 20 percent symptomatic patients at that point would indeed indicate more serious underlying pathology or at least warrant further investigation.

Sinusitis

Topic. Another health problem selected for study was sinusitis, with emphasis on the health outcomes of therapeutic management. The provider group was again a university health maintenance organization in a small, newly developed town in a county adjacent to a large metropolis. The patient population consisted of consecutive adult clinic walk-ins with a current diagnosis of sinusitis; their average age was 33 (range, 18 to 55), and 64 females and 40 males of middle class background were involved. The topic was selected because it is common, produces moderate distress and disability, and can usually be treated successfully.

Design. Sampling was prospective to yield approximately 100 consecutive clinic walk-ins with a diagnosis of sinusitis. Health outcomes were to be measured at the end of a three to four week interval by means of a standard questionnaire administered by telephone (mail in 5 cases). A chart review was undertaken at the same time to determine other illnesses, laboratory results, treatments, and previous episodes of this problem. Final outcomes were correlated with patient compliance, previous episodes, allergies, smoking, and nose surgery. Patient satisfaction with care was also measured. Health outcome standards developed by the clinic study team indicated that if more than 34 percent of the study sample were symptomatic at followup, further inquiry into outcome determinants would be warranted.

Results. Of the 104 patients in the sample, complete data were collected for 100, for a 96 percent response rate. As shown in Table 8.10, measured health outcomes were significantly worse than maximum acceptable standards. Subsequent analysis conducted to identify correctable determinants of the deficiency led to the identification of two prognostic subgroups, of which one had no negative prognostic factors, while the second group had a history of allergy, smoked one or more packs of cigarettes a day, or were immunologically compromised, e.g., due to being on steroids or having diabetes mellitus. It appeared that half of the better prognostic group and two-thirds of the worse group were still symptomatic and required further management three to four weeks following diagnosis. There were no other

Table 8.10. Health care assessment results in a study of sinusitis in adults

Provider Characteristics	Patient and Sample Characteristics	Therapeutic Outcomes (as percent at each level)		Sample Size (n) and Completion Rate (percent)	
		Obs***	MAS	n	%
Study 14 Facility 5					
Prepaid university HMO in an eastern town in a metropolitan region. 45 physicians	Middle class adults. Prospective sampling of consecutive walk-in patients diagnosed as having sinusitis; 3–4 week followup	(n = 100) Asymptomatic, normal and high risk		104	96
		38	65		
		Symptomatic 61	34		
		Restricted 1	1		
		Dependent 0	0		
		Dead 0	0		

***P < 0.001

correlations of significance when health outcomes were related to compliance, previous episodes, nose surgery, allergies, and smoking.

However, several minor management deficiencies were noted, i.e., five patients were given antibiotics without previous cultures; in two cases, throat rather than nasal cultures were done; and two patients were not contacted when cultures revealed that an inappropriate antibiotic had been prescribed. The main problem seemed to be a lack of adequate followup to check patient health status and identify continued symptomatology.

A satisfaction questionnaire indicated that 43 percent were highly satisfied with care, 20 percent were satisfied and had no complaints, and 34 percent had one or more complaints.

Implications. This outcome study revealed a slightly neglected health problem in terms of prolonged symptoms. The fact that patient lifestyle was disrupted in only 1 percent of the cases studied probably indicates adequate management overall. In the absence of positive correlations with compliance and other disease factors, it is questionable whether much more could have been done to lower the percentage of patients who were symptomatic after three or four weeks. However, a question regarding the priority judgment of the clinical staff might be raised. It seems debatable whether or not there was a significant amount of preventable health impairment related to sinusitis that was not being prevented at the clinic. The finding also raises the question of whether health outcome standards should have been less stringent in this case. The significant symptom level at three to four weeks after diagnosis was not clearly attributable to inadequate care. Extending the followup interval to eight weeks would perhaps have facilitated more meaningful assessment results, as patients symptomatic after that time would certainly require further investigation. On the other hand, the failure of this group to plan and implement improvement actions and to reevaluate the results would indicate that the staff may not have judged the benefits to be worth the effort.

Vaginitis

Topic. The health problem selected for study in a fee for service and prepaid clinic in the Midwest was acute or chronic inflammation of the vulva or vagina due either to specific causes, i.e., monilia, gonorrhea, trichomoniasis, or herpes, or any nonspecific cause. The physicians were primarily staff gynecologists, though five patients were seen in family practice and one in an internal medicine clinic.

The patient population consisted of late adolescent (including many college students) and adult women primarily diagnosed in the clinic. The study focus was on the outcomes of therapeutic management.

Design. The study was based on prospective sampling for approximately 100 consecutive walk-in patients receiving a diagnosis of vulva, vaginal, or vulva-vaginal inflammation; atrophic vaginitis; or nonspecific vaginitis. Patients were given a standard health questionnaire on symptom recurrence and on antibiotics and contraceptives taken. At the same time, a chart review was conducted to identify associated health problems and treatments given, including contraceptives. A followup study was conducted by questionnaire ten months following the initial diagnosis. Assessment standards developed by the clinic study team indicated that if less than 85 percent of the study sample were not fully recovered one month following treatment, further inquiry would be considered necessary.

Results. Although a total of 112 patients qualified for study, complete followup data were obtained from only 42. As shown in Table 8.11, the ten month followup results indicated that over half of the patients had experienced a treatment failure, well over maximum acceptable standards.

Subsequent analysis revealed that 24 of the 42 patients responding were on oral contraceptives and that, as expected, monilial infections predominated in this group (18); only 8 of the 24 experienced recovery with no return of the symptoms. The study team recognized lack of generalizability of results due to the poor response rate, but it did examine correctable factors in the group for which data were available. In the total group of 42, 17 of the patients proved to have inadequate understanding regarding instructions about taking medication. Most discontinued therapy early, mainly when menstruation started or when it became inconvenient. The study team estimated that inadequate understanding accounted for at least 40 percent of the treatment failure. None of the 8 patients having trichomonous infection had their sexual partners checked for this infection. The observed failure rate was highest for the total group of monilial infections (16 out of 27) and slightly lower for the trichomonous group (4 out of 8) and the nonspecific group (4 out of 7).

Implications. Therapeutic outcomes were far below standards in this study, and the length of time over which these women suffered symptoms underscores the importance of this problem. There would seem to be much that could have been done by way of improved management, especially as related to patient education and followup care.

The quality assurance implications of this study relate primarily to the inadequate response rate. It should be noted, however, that this topic was part of an initial set of studies conducted in this clinic, and it did serve the purpose of sensitizing staff to the problems involved in achieving better response rates. Also, this was one of the studies where the standard health scale was not applied, although it was specified in the original design. While it is unlikely that this particular medical problem produced serious disruption of patient life in terms of work or self-care activities, an overall measure reflecting quality of life and functional ability is an important routine measure. Also, though important correctable determinants of the deficient outcomes were identified, no subsequent improvement action was taken in this project.

Penicillin and Infectious Disease

Topic. Two clinics elected to cooperate in a study of outcomes of penicillin utilization in relation to infectious disease, specifically, the unnecessary prescription of penicillin by the staff. The providers were primary care physicians in two adjacent health maintenance organizations in a western metropolis, and patients in the two clinics were pooled for sampling purposes; the population consisted of working class patients. Both diagnostic and therapeutic outcomes were assessed.

Design. A retrospective, consecutive two month sample was drawn from the sample frame of all walk-in patients seen in the two clinics. The assessment measure was a chart review form to be completed for all patients with a penicillin prescription in their medical records. The records were also screened for all diagnoses and recorded results of any smears or cultures and sensitivity tests. Table 8.12 lists indications for penicillin utilization as stipulated by the study team.

A one in four sample of patients was contacted one month after treatment for a personal interview to determine overall health status in terms of the six level health and disability scale (see Chapter 6). Assessment standards were defined by the clinic study team in terms of the maximum acceptable rate of unnecessary penicillin use, as well as of maximum group disability after one month.

Results. Charts for 6,572 walk-in patients in the two month study interval were reviewed. Although 6 percent of the charts, a

Table 8.11.   Health care assessment results in a study of vaginitis in adolescent and adult females

Provider Characteristics	Patient and Sample Characteristics	Therapeutic Outcomes^a (as percent at each level)	Obs***	MAS	Sample Size (n) and Completion Rate (percent) n	%
Study 32 Facility 10						
Fee for service and prepaid clinic in a midwestern rural town. 16 physicians	Middle and working class females (adolescent and adult). Prospective sampling of walk-in patients diagnosed as having vaginitis; 10 month followup	(n = 42) Recovery	45	85	112	38
		Treatment failure— 1 month	33	12		
		Treatment failure— 2-3 months	14	2		
		Treatment failure— 4-10 months	7	0		

^{a}Health problem outcomes; overall health outcomes not assessed.
***P < 0.001

Table 8.12. Indications for penicillin utilization in a study of diagnostic and therapeutic outcomes

Study 48		
Qualifying Organisms[a]	Smears/Cultures	Qualifying Diagnoses
Beta hemolytic streptococcus	Pneumococci	Cellulitis
Staphylococcus aureus coagulase (+)	Meningococci	Erysipelas
If penicillin sensitive	Treponemia pallidum	Carbuncles Furuncles Impetigo

[a]Penicillin given prior to culture report acceptable.

total of 410, indicated that penicillin had been prescribed during the two month period, cultures and sensitivities had been reported in only 18 percent (69 cases), and in 35 percent of these, the organism was insensitive to penicillin. Of the 410 having penicillin prescribed, therefore, use of this drug was unsupportable by staff standards for 84 percent, as shown in Table 8.13.

From the one in four sample of 100 patients on penicillin drawn for followup interview, 96 completed questionnaires were obtained, for a response rate of 96 percent. Here, the results revealed the overall health status of the group to be well within standards.

The study team examined the direct financial implications of this apparent penicillin overutilization. While the average cost of penicillin prescribed was approximately $3 per person (1972 dollars), the cost of a culture and sensitivity was $12 per person. Extrapolation to a full year would indicate that 2,460 patients might receive penicillin at a cost of $7,380, but that if all of these patients were to receive cultures and sensitivity tests, total costs would be $29,520. Assuming, again by extrapolation, that 35 percent grew organisms insensitive to penicillin, $29,520 would have had to be spent in order to save $2,583 in unnecessary penicillin cost. Consequently, the health risks of giving unnecessary penicillin must be weighed against the apparent economic savings of not ordering cultures and sensitivity tests routinely.

Implications. The clinical implications of this study are somewhat controversial. The convention in these two clinics is probably widespread: prescribe penicillin now, read culture results later—if cultures are ordered at all. The findings indicate that if cultures are in fact

Table 8.13. Health care assessment results in a study of penicillin utilization in adults and children

Provider Characteristics	Patient and Sample Characteristics	Diagnostic Outcomes[a] (as percent in each category)		Therapeutic Outcomes (as percent at each level)		Sample Size (n) and Completion Rate (percent)			
						Diagnostic		Therapeutic	
		Obs	MAS	Obs	MAS	n	%	n	%
Study 48 Facility 19 and 20									
Prepaid HMO in western metropolitan region. 21 physicians	Working class adults and children. Retrospective 2 month sampling of consecutive charts for patients receiving prescriptions for penicillin; 1 month followup of one in four subsample of those on penicillin	(n = 410) False positives 84***	5	(n = 96)		410	100	100	96
				Asymptomatic, normal risk 48	8				
				Asymptomatic, high risk 0	27				
				Symptomatic 44	51				
				Restricted 3	3				
				Dependent 5	10				
				Dead 0	1				

[a]False positives defined as no indication for penicillin utilization by staff standards.
***P < 0.001

ordered, there may be a two in three chance of being correct in prescribing penicillin. On the other hand, the staff members of this clinic had indicated through their study team that no more than 5 percent of cases of penicillin use should be unsupported by identification of a penicillin sensitive organism proven by cultures; suggested by smears; or presumed by diagnosis of several limited conditions (usually skin infections), where such use was considered justified without cultures.

The staff's own performance indicated that 84 percent of their penicillin prescriptions would not meet their own list of indications, mainly due to lack of tests to identify the organism. On the other hand, the economic implications of routine ordering of cultures and sensitivity or other available tests were high, increasing costs of care for these patients as a group by a factor of four. This is a quandary that can best be resolved by research documentation of the probable health implications of unnecessary penicillin use. What is the proportion of patients receiving unnecessary penicillin who might have an anaphylactic reaction? Current estimates place this figure at around 10 to 40 per 100,000 injections (Dershewitz, 1977). How many in what age groups are likely to die from this or other complications? What proportion will be harmed by altered bacterial flora in their body? How many will develop penicillin resistant strains that may later infect them or those whom they contact? These are serious questions that require documented answers.

There are some conditions where a culture might be crucial—for example, sore throats in children and young adults. Conversely, there are some conditions where penicillin is probably futile, as in uncomplicated upper respiratory tract virus infections without pharyngitis or in allergies. The profile of such problems may have to be examined in each clinic to determine the relative proportion of clear indications for and against penicillin use.

The quality assurance implications of this study, on the other hand, are clear. Unless the efficacy of treatment and prognoses in terms of risk with and without treatment are established, effort on assessment measurements will be rather futile. Ending a time consuming study with more questions raised than answered may be acceptable in research, but is of limited utility in care evaluation. Quality assessment studies must be designed to yield clear-cut directions for subsequent improvement action. In this study, this was not accomplished, primarily because of the failure to do a literature search or to establish consensus on achievable benefit, and consequently assessment implications are controversial at best.

ENDOCRINE DISEASE—
DIABETES MELLITUS

Diabetes mellitus was the only endocrine disease studied in this phase of the health accounting project; it was selected as a topic in four different institutions. Again, the importance of therapeutic outcomes and the relative ease of establishing a diagnosis probably contributed to the choice.

Topic

Diabetes mellitus was the study topic in four institutions, where the providers were primary care physicians in three multispecialty group practices and one hospital. Two of the groups were fee for service, and one a prepaid health maintenance organization. In two instances (the hospital and one clinic), the population selected for study were patients with measured fasting blood sugars; in the other two facilities, consecutive walk-in patients were screened. Two patient groups were mixed middle and working class; one, working class; and one, poverty class. The focus of assessment was diagnostic outcomes in one study, both diagnostic and therapeutic outcomes in another, and therapeutic outcomes only in two studies.

Design

In the two diagnostic screening studies, the design was retrospective. In the hospital study of consecutive admissions (Study 3), a chart review was completed for all patients having had routine admission screening fasting blood sugar in excess of 130 mg%. If no evidence of a diagnosis of diabetes or of any physician mention, repeat test, or other relevant response to the high blood sugar levels was found, the patient was labeled a false negative or missed diagnosis.

In Study 42, a six month retrospective sample of all clinic walk-in patients over age 35 without a previous diagnosis of diabetes was studied. A chart review was undertaken to identify all patients who met one or more of thirteen indications for diabetic screening, e.g., strong family history, overweight, or previous routine fasting blood sugar test results in excess of 120 mg%. Again, if no physician mention of possible diabetes, repeat test, or other relevant response was found, the patient was classified as a false negative. If the patient had not required diabetic screening by these criteria but received a blood sugar test, he was considered a false positive.

In the three therapeutic outcome studies, a followup patient interview or mailout questionnaire was completed by patients diagnosed

Table 8.14. Prognostic weights for patients with diabetes mellitus

	Study 34		Study 39	
	Prognosis		Prognostic Factor	Prognostic Weight
	Favorable	Unfavorable		
Age of onset < 40 years				
Duration	20 years or less	More than 20 years	Duration ≥ 10 years	3
			< 12 years	1
Insulin-dependent	No	Yes	Age of onset ≥ 30	3
			< 30	1
Weight	Normal	Abnormal	Insulin dependent	4
Regular medical care	Yes	No	Insulin independent	2
On welfare	No	Yes	Complications	5
Complications	No	Yes	Uropathy	5
Primary disease	No	Yes	Neuropathy	1
Family history	No	Yes	Retinopathy	3
Age of onset > 40 years			Associated Disease	
Duration	10 years or less	More than 10 years	Cardiovascular	4
Insulin dependent	No	Yes	Obesity	1
Weight	Normal or less	Abnormally high	Malignancy	5
Regular medical care	—	Yes	Best prognosis	0-5
On welfare	No	Yes	Intermediate prognosis	5-10
Complications	No	Yes	Worst prognosis	> 10
Primary disease	No	Yes		
Family history	No	Yes		

—Not recorded.

as "diabetic" (Studies 34 and 39) or as "adult onset diabetic" (Study 42). The followup periods ranged from four months to one year. In Studies 34 and 39, the patients were further divided into three prognostic groups—poor, average, and best—using a set of weighted prognostic factors (Table 8.14). Health outcomes were calculated separately for each of these groups. Additional demographic and related medical information was compiled for both Studies 34 and 39 (Table 8.15), and in Study 34, a special inquiry was made with respect to patients who had died during the followup interval.

Maximum acceptable standards both in terms of the percentage of missed diagnoses or false negatives (and misdiagnoses or false positives for Study 42) and of acceptable outcomes were established by each study team to indicate the extent of deficiency that could be tolerated before further inquiry would be made.

Results

Assessment of diagnostic outcomes revealed that serious diabetic suspects were being missed in 91 percent (Study 3) and 13 percent (Study 42) of the cases (Table 8.16). Tests were unwarranted by study criteria in 23 percent of the cases in Study 42, which assessed false positives as well. All three results were significantly different from the maximum acceptable standards of 1, 5, and 15 percent, respectively. In Study 3, the performance deficiency was correlated neither with the severity of the blood sugar level nor with physician specialty; an exception was surgery, where performance was significantly worse than for all other physicians. The number of years in practice was directly related to deficient outcomes.

Therapeutic outcomes were significantly worse than acceptable in two instances (Studies 34 and 42) and within standards in one (Study 39). Analysis of the 10 deaths (9 percent) in Study 34 revealed that the median age of the deceased patients was 66, with a range from 55 to 80. Three patients died of causes remote from diabetes mellitus (chronic lymphatic leukemia, carcinoma of the pancreas, and pulmonary emphysema). The remaining seven died of cerebral or cardiovascular lesions or of infections that could well have been directly related to diabetes mellitus, which was severe in all seven cases. Overall, the staff judged that these deaths were not preventable, basing this conclusion on the fact that each of the ten had received close medical attention prior to death and had complied reasonably well with the management provided.

In Study 39, patient management outcomes were considered seriously deficient: 27 percent were not on a diet; 54 percent of those on a diet were not adhering to it; and 14 percent were not seeing a

Table 8.15.   Percentage distribution of medical management and demographic factors among patients followed for diabetes mellitus in two outcome assessment studies

As percent in each category

Medical and Demographic Factors	Study 34 (n = 117)	Study 39 (n = 135)	Management and Demographic Factors	Study 34 (n = 117)	Study 39 (n = 135)
Duration of diabetes			Management		
Nine years average duration	50		Sees physician regularly	—	86
Ten years average duration		81	On diabetic diet	—	73
Type of diabetes			Follows diet well	—	46
Insulin dependent	26	25	Diet only treatment	4	—
Insulin independent	74	75	Oral antidiabetics	54	61
Complications			Insulin	36	26
Diabetic, uropathy	9	15	Admitted to hospital in past six months	29	23
Diabetic, neuropathy	3	30	Hospitalized for diabetes in past six months	—	10
Diabetic, retinopathy	9	27	Had to see eye doctor in past six months	—	30
Cataracts	8	—	Demography		
Obesity	49	—	Mean age	53	—
Cardiovascular	48	67	Male	35	—
Heart disease	—	34	Middle class	26	—
Hypertension	—	41	Working class	64	—
Kidney disease	—	18	Poverty class	10	—
Cancer	1	11	Family history of diabetes mellitus	43	—
Pyelonephritis in past six months	—	14			

—Not applicable.

physician regularly (see Table 8.15). Health problem outcomes were equally questionable; 61 percent of patients not on insulin were taking oral hypoglycemics; 23 percent had been hospitalized in the past six months, 10 percent of these for diabetes; 14 percent had developed kidney infections in the past six months; and 30 percent had vision problems in this period.

Implications

The clinical implications of the diagnostic deficiencies depend upon how much health benefit or harm is judged possible for treating the predominant group found, i.e., insulin independent diabetics. Many now consider this problem controversial at best. If subsequent clinical research continues to reinforce the findings of the University Group Diabetes Program (1970), the detection of these patients could even be damaging if oral antidiabetics are prescribed as indiscriminately as they seem to be at present. Of the total diabetic population in Studies 34 and 39, 54 and 61 percent, respectively, were found to be on these drugs. Whether or not the high death rate in Study 34 (9 percent) was related to previous inadequate care, use of oral antidiabetics, or other correctable deficiencies is not clear and in any event was denied by the staff.

In all three therapeutic outcome studies (Studies 34, 39, 42), analysis of the patients with severe disability revealed that their diabetes was, in most cases, related directly to the degree of overall disability measured. The teams were far less negative about the preventability of impairment found (e.g., polineuritis, trophic ulcers, retinopathy). It would seem that more specific consideration of each patient will be necessary for more definitive clinical judgments.

The quality assurance implications are more clear-cut. The need for a more rigorously documented basis for establishing attribution of health outcomes to medical care provided or neglected is borne out in this study. The University Group Diabetes Study provides the most definitive evidence on this subject in relation to complications of asymptomatic, insulin independent diabetes (Goldner, Knatterud, and Prout, 1971; University Group Diabetes Program, 1970). It was found that strict blood sugar control by use of oral antidiabetics or insulin had little relationship to any of the complications observed. On the other hand, blood sugar control in insulin dependent diabetes has more convincing evidence to indicate reduced target organ disease (Cahill, Ertzwiler, and Freinkel, 1976). In this latter group especially, there may be considerable preventable impairment in terms of symptoms and hospitalization episodes if patient health

Table 8.16.   Health care assessment results in four studies of diabetes mellitus in adults

Provider Characteristics	Patient and Sample Characteristics	Diagnostic Outcomes (as percent in each category)		Therapeutic Outcomes (as percent at each level)		Sample Size (n) and Completion Rate (percent)			
						Diagnostic		Therapeutic	
		Obs	MAS	Obs **	MAS	n	%	n	%
Study 3 Facility 1									
Fee for service community hospital in a midwestern city. 114 physicians	Middle and working class adults. Retrospective consecutive sample (1 year) of hospital admissions routinely screened for FBSb > 130 mg%	(n = 122) False negatives[a] 91	*** 1			4175	100		
Study 34 Facility 11									
Multispecialty private fee for service clinic in a midwestern town. 29 physicians	Working and middle class adults. Retrospective-prospective (6 months) consecutive sample of patients suspected of diabetes on the basis of laboratory test reports indicating FBSb > 120 mg%; 1 year followup			(n = 117) Asymptomatic, normal and high risk 46; Symptomatic 35; Restricted 8; Dependent 3; Dead 9	59; 26; 8; 5; 2			132	89

Study 39 Facility 13

Multispecialty private fee for service clinic in a rural south central town. 50 physicians

Working class adults. Prospective sample (7 months) of consecutive walk-in patients diagnosed as diabetic; 6 month followup

(n = 135)	Obs	MAS	n	%
Asymptomatic, normal and high risk	47	46		
Symptomatic	37	20		
Restricted	10	18		
Dependent	5	8		
Dead	1	7	150	90

Study 42 Facility 14

Multispecialty prepaid HMO in western metropolitan region 13 physicians

Poverty class adults. Retrospective chart review for patients over 35 years seen within 6 months and not previously diagnosed as diabetic. 4 month followup of one-in-two sample of patients with FBS[b] > 120 mg%

	Obs	MAS
(n = 173) False negatives[c]	13***	5
(n = 195) False positives[c]	23**	15

(n = 105)	Obs***	MAS	n	%	n	%
Asymptomatic, normal risk	0	0				
Asymptomatic, high risk	18	60				
Symptomatic	20	9				
Restricted	49	20				
Dependent	11	6				
Dead	2	6	1033	99	126	83

[a]False negatives refer to absence of diagnosis of diabetes mellitus or further diabetic screening despite initial elevated blood sugar or other indication.

[b]FBS = fasting blood sugar.

[c]Diagnostic screening outcomes, where false negatives refer to absence of diabetes screening despite screening indications and false positives to screening tests performed in the absence of positive indications.

 **P < 0.01

***P < 0.001

education is improved. A literature survey would seem essential in planning future studies on this topic.

Although the maximum acceptable standards developed varied widely from study to study, subsequent evaluation revealed substantive reasons for these differences and supported their validity. In Study 39, with the least stringent standards, the staff were prepared to tolerate almost one-third of their patients unable to work, bedridden, or dead. The large amount of concomitant nondiabetic disease (e.g., 11 percent of their patients had cancer) may have justified this. On the other hand, the standards in Study 34 indicated the staff to be twice as stringent, focusing as they were on diabetic suspects, i.e., patients in a much earlier stage of their disease. It was held that if more than 15 percent of this group were found to be unable to work, bedridden, or dead, a more detailed inquiry into correctable causes would be indicated. Although all four study teams proceeded to the definitive assessment stage of the health accounting strategy (see Chapter 6), none implemented improvement action.

NEOPLASTIC DISEASE

Topic
Neoplasms were the health problem selected for four studies in three clinics. Two focused on carcinoma of the prostate, one on basal cell skin carcinoma, and one on breast cancer. All providers were on the staff of multispecialty fee for service clinics and were mainly urologists and surgeons. The patient population consisted of middle and working class patients with diagnosed carcinoma recorded in their medical records. The assessment focus was on therapeutic outcomes, measured at followup intervals as indicated by each condition.

Design
In three of the studies, the sample was selected by review of the tumor registry (Study 13), patient charts (Study 22) or operative records (Study 12) until approximately 100 patients had been accumulated. In Study 25, the tumor registry was searched for all patients diagnosed within one year for cancer of the prostate. Every patient in the sample was contacted either by phone, by mail, or in person to complete a standard health status questionnaire rating each subject at one of six levels of the standard health scale. In Studies 12 and 13, a patient satisfaction questionnaire was also administered.

Maximum acceptable standards were developed by the clinic study teams, which were composed of staff physicians knowledgeable with regard to the carcinoma being investigated. In each instance, the standard was a theoretical distribution of 100 patients on the six level health status scale representing the maximum group disability the clinic team could accept without further inquiry.

In all studies, weighted prognostic correlates were developed to facilitate more detailed analysis of health outcomes by controlling for severity. The prognostic factors usually included patient age, stage and grade of the carcinoma, and the presence of complications or other serious disease. For example, in Study 13 (basal cell carcinoma of the skin), the following simple weighting scale was developed to indicate two prognostic groups, the best prognostic group having less than four points and the worst group five or more:

Factor	Weight
First time tumor treated	1
Recurrent when treated	3
Located in area of eyes, nose, ears	2
Other locations	1
Basisquamous cell	2
Basal cell	1

Results

As shown in Table 8.17, maximum acceptable disability was exceeded in both carcinoma of the prostate studies, but not in the basal cell skin and breast carcinoma groups.

In Study 22, subsequent inquiry was conducted to identify correctable determinants of the seemingly deficient outcomes. A review of the 33 deaths (38 percent) revealed the following causes of death:

Carcinoma of the prostate	16
Other carcinoma	2
Cardiac disease	4
Cerebrovascular accident	1
Pneumonitis	1
Unknown	9

While all of the patients whose deaths were attributable to prostate carcinoma had been in advanced stages, there was serious concern that the other deaths might have been a result of the urologist acting as the primary physician and providing poorer general care. This was not found to be a problem in this sample; each patient had been closely followed by an internist or general practitioner. The only correctable factors identified were failure to study renal function in 16 percent and the possible use of radiation and orchiectomy for patients with Stage C carcinoma. The clinic study team claimed that there

Table 8.17.   Health care assessment results in four studies of neoplasms in adults

Provider Characteristics	Patient and Sample Characteristics	Therapeutic Outcomes (as percent at each level)		Sample Size (n) and Completion Rate (percent)	
		Obs	MAS	n	%
Study 12 Facility 4					
Private multi-specialty fee for service clinic in a midwestern metropolis. 26 physicians	Middle and working class females. Retrospective sampling of consecutive women operated for breast cancer over 10 year period; 3–13 year followup	(n = 82)		89	92
	Asymptomatic, normal and high risk	20	26		
	Symptomatic	23	11		
	Restricted	12	4		
	Dependent	5	0		
	Dead	40	59		
Study 13 Facility 4		Obs	MAS	n	%
Private multi-specialty fee for service clinic in a midwestern metropolis. 26 physicians	Middle and working class adults. Retrospective sampling of consecutive patients in tumor registry with basal cell skin carcinoma; 3–7 year followup	(n = 84)		100	84
	Asymptomatic, normal and high risk	91	79		
	Symptomatic	5	20		
	Restricted	0	0		
	Dependent	0	0		
	Dead	4	0		

Study 22 Facility 8

Private multi-specialty fee for service and prepaid clinic in rural eastern town. 197 physicians

Working class males. Retrospective chart review (1 year) for consecutive patients with cancer of the prostate; 18 month followup

(n = 86)	Obs***	MAS	n	%
Asymptomatic, normal risk	2	5	100	86
Asymptomatic, high risk	10	11		
Symptomatic	25	33		
Restricted	21	22		
Dependent	4	12		
Dead	38	17		

Study 25 Facility 9

Private multi-specialty fee for service clinic in rural midwestern town. 115 physicians

Middle and working class males. Retrospective sampling (1 year) of all patients in tumor registry with cancer of the prostate; 2 year followup

(n = 50)	Obs *	MAS	n	%
Asymptomatic, normal and high risk	12	20	52	96
Symptomatic	36	42		
Restricted	16	16		
Dependent	14	12		
Dead	22	10		

*P < 0.05
***P < 0.001

was a dramatic linear relationship between the prognostic weights and the health scale levels measured and stated that the factors included seemed to be highly significant in terms of predicting overall disability.

In Study 25, despite a death rate twice that considered acceptable, no further analysis was conducted, due primarily to physician skepticism about the assessment method. The standards were considered to have little meaning. When it was pointed out how closely the measured health scale distributions reflected a previous study in that clinic of 600 patients with carcinoma of the prostate, the staff claimed that there must have been poor sampling in the study or other procedural flaws explaining the seemingly deficient results.

In Study 12, the most interesting finding was the unexpected longevity of this group of breast cancer patients, which was well within acceptable standards. There was concern about the higher than expected percentage of patients who were symptomatic or away from major life activity (Table 8.18). Most of these patients had had a radical as opposed to a simple mastectomy, and nearly two out of three having radical surgery had serious postoperative complications

Table 8.18. Therapeutic outcomes for breast cancer patients by prognostic group

	Study 12							
Therapeutic Outcomes (as percent at each level)	Diagnostic Prognosis				Treatment Prognosis			
	Best[a] (n = 39)		Worst[b] (n = 37)		Best[c] (n = 29)		Worst[d] (n = 53)	
	Obs	MAS	Obs	MAS	Obs	MAS	Obs	MAS
Asymptomatic, normal and high risk	36	58	5	9	45	58	6	9
Symptomatic	23	20	24	6	24	20	23	6
Restricted	21	2	8	5	17	2	9	5
Dependent	5	0	3	0	4	0	6	0
Dead	15	20	60	80	10	20	56	80

[a]Axillary lymph nodes not involved.
[b]Axillary lymph nodes involved.
[c]Without radiation.
[d]With radiation.

Note: Six patients were excluded from diagnostic prognosis assessment because lymph node involvement was not determined.

that slowed convalescence. A special meeting of the surgeons was held to review all of these patients. They concluded that the extent of the incision and the resulting complications were responsible for the extensive disability in this group. Even more important, as a result of this study the surgeons recognized that they had previously judged operative success only by lack of subsequent disease. They became convinced that they should be more sensitive to subsequent patient functioning, which might be improved by less extensive surgery and more attention to postoperative physiotherapy. Despite resulting complications and disability, on the other hand, the patients expressed general satisfaction with the care received.

In Study 13, observed findings on basal cell skin carcinoma outcomes showed no significant departure from standards, with the exception of a 4 percent unexpected death rate. However, subsequent inquiry into correctable determinants of this mortality showed that all deaths were related to old age and not to the carcinoma, regardless of prognostic grouping. An interesting sidelight was the fact that here, too, patients were satisfied with the care received and were markedly uninterested in the cosmetic effects of their treatment, possibly due to old age. The physicians on the team concluded that they might be even more thorough in their treatment in the future.

Implications

The clinical implications of these studies of carcinoma were disappointing. No dramatic health improvement seemed achievable by altering patient management, with the exception of the breast cancer group, where significant potential for improved patient comfort and functional status by altered surgical techniques would seem possible.

The quality assurance implications of these studies were mixed. As mentioned before, one group (Study 25) was not at all impressed with the assessment approach applied and took no further action in this instance. It is of interest, though, that the same staff later voted to include outcome assessment methods as a permanent approach in their ongoing medical audit program. This action may have been due to the enthusiasm of the quality assurance coordinator, however. The three remaining groups did accept this approach from the outset and were motivated to study the results in more detail, making recommendations for improvement in two instances.

Of special interest were the overly pessimistic standards set for breast cancer outcomes, that is, a 59 percent case fatality rate for a three to thirteen year followup interval. While a finding of only 40 percent deaths was encouraging, the serious functional disability found in the total group of patients remained statistically insignificant because the acceptable rate of deaths had been set so high. However, subsequent analysis was to lead to an important educational outcome; the surgeons involved seemed to alter their attitude toward functional outcomes substantially and seemed to be placing greater value on the patient as a person. They altered surgical technique and emphasized rehabilitation in order to improve postoperative patient comfort and function, whereas previously they had been primarily interested in longevity and the prevention of recurrence of the neoplasm. Subsequent outcome standards set by this group will probably reflect more realistically what they have learned and underscore the potential for self-correction of this quality assurance approach.

CARDIOVASCULAR AND CEREBROVASCULAR DISEASE

Topic
Four clinics elected to study lesions involving the vasculature of the brain and heart (i.e., emboli, thrombi, and hemorrhage). Two projects related to initial cerebrovascular accidents and two to myocardial infarctions, with one focusing on the complication of heart failure.

The providers were university faculty and house staff in two studies and private fee for service clinic staff in the other two. Three studies involved mainly internists or family physicians, while physiatrists from a university department of physical medicine and rehabilitation comprised most of the fourth study team.

The patient populations studied ranged from middle and working class to poverty populations and included both males and females. Both studies of cerebrovascular accidents centered on specific age groups; in Study 35, 78 percent of the patients were aged 65 to 85 or above; and in Study 57, an arbitrary age limit of 60 was set, the mean age of the sample being 45. The focus of study was on both diagnostic and therapeutic outcomes in Study 9 and on therapeutic outcomes only in Studies 19, 35, and 57.

Design
One study of myocardial infarction (Study 9) prospectively sampled consecutive admissions to the hospital coronary care unit from the emergency room during a six month interval. The remaining three used retrospective sampling by reviewing medical records until a series of approximately 100 patients with a relevant recorded

diagnosis had been collected. In Study 19, only hospitalized patients referred back to their clinic physician were included.

For purposes of the diagnostic outcome study of hospitalized myocardial infarction suspects (Study 9), a chart review was conducted in relation to forty items of history, physical examination, or laboratory information related to the diagnosis of congestive heart failure. For 113 of 122 patients in the sample, the recorded information was sufficiently complete for an independent study team to make a diagnosis. The diagnosis made by the attending physicians (either recorded or implied by therapy ordered) was likewise determined and compared to diagnoses of the independent study team. False negatives (missed diagnoses) or false positives (misdiagnoses) were tabulated, and the rates were compared to maximum acceptable standards developed by the medical staff.

In the second study of myocardial infarction (Study 19), patients were included in the sample only if they had chest pain, characteristic enzyme elevations, and/or electrocardiographic changes reflecting damage of the myocardium. Each patient was also assigned to a "good" and "poor" prognostic group, based on the following scale:

Previous myocardial infarction	20
Acute complications (e.g., shock)	20
Extensive myocardial infarction	10
Diastolic pressure > 100 mm Hg	10
Metabolic defect (e.g., increased cholesterol, diabetes mellitus, or uric acid)	10
Age < 40 or > 65	10
Persistent angina	10
Family history of arteriosclerotic heart disease	5
Cigarette smoking	5

Scores of 20 points or less were considered a good prognosis, and separate health outcome standards were developed for each prognostic subgroup, as well as for the group as a whole.

In Study 35, the staff did not specify case selection criteria other than a recorded diagnosis of cerebrovascular accident, although two prognostic groups of the patients in the sample were identified based on psychosocial and economic factors, primary disease, paralysis, speech impairment, and type and location of lesion. Separate impairment standards were set for each group.

In Study 57, the following criteria were applied:

- Stroke must be patient's first;
- Patient must have been hospitalized for at least three weeks;
- Chart must have a diagnosis of hemiparesis, hemiplegia, and/or aphasia for 48 hours or more; and
- Chart must indicate a suspected or confirmed thrombosis, hemorrhage, aneurysm, or embolism.

Also, a modification of the standard health scale was used in Study 57 (see Table 8.19), which expanded levels 3, 4, and 5 of the standard scale to make it more sensitive to the functional disability of the stroke group by including self-care and major activity ratings. For this purpose, an additional questionnaire was developed by the study team to measure changes in function related to ambulation, social and psychological adjustment, and communication.

In all four therapeutic outcome assessments, the patients were contacted by phone, mail, or personal interview to apply the standard health status questionnaire. The followup interval, from time of initial diagnosis, ranged from three to thirteen years in Study 57 to approximately one year in Studies 9 and 19.

Results

The assessment of diagnostic outcomes in Study 9 in relation to heart failure in acute coronary suspects revealed no significant discrepancy between observed rates and acceptable standards. The rates of false negative and false positive diagnoses were 3 percent and 0 percent, respectively (Table 8.19). The health outcome assessment for the same group of patients measured one year later also revealed no overall significant deviation from standards. However, on noting an unusually high proportion (23 percent) of patients not back to their usual life activity (gainful employment in nearly all cases), the staff conducted an additional inquiry into this group. The surprising finding was that nearly two out of three of these patients were acute myocardial infarction suspects who when hospitalized had been found not to have had a myocardial infarction. (Over 60 percent of patients admitted to this coronary care unit for observation are usually found to have noncardiac causes of their chest pain or distress.) As a result of this study, arrangements were made for routine postdischarge followup of coronary care unit patients. Subsequently, vocational rehabilitation counseling was stressed. A followup outcome assessment study was planned but has not been implemented.

In the other study of myocardial infarction (Study 19), however, the assessment of health outcomes revealed a significant deviation from standards. There were more deaths and more patients restricted from major life activity than acceptable. Further analysis by splitting the total sample into the previously established "good" and "poor" prognostic groups revealed the surprising finding that the major discrepancy between observed health outcomes and standards had occurred in the good prognostic group of 36 patients, as shown in Table 8.20. There were fewer asymptomatic patients, more still away from major life activity (usually vocational work), and more dead than acceptable. The same analysis for the 44 patients in the poor prognostic group revealed measured findings well within standards, however. Consequently, further inquiry was made regarding both the total "restricted" group in this study and the deaths. A brief review revealed no clear explanation for the death and disability measured, which certainly was not explained by cardiac pathology. Analysis revealed that 19 of the 34 deaths occurred on initial hospitalization. Of the remaining 15, 11 died six months to one year later. Unfortunately, causes of death were not recorded. In the judgment of the staff, no correctable determinants of deficiency could be found to warrant improvement action.

Health outcome assessment in the first stroke study (Study 35) likewise revealed a clear discrepancy between observed findings and standards. Subsequent analysis by prognostic groups revealed that the major discrepancy was in the poor prognostic group constituted by 80 out of the 86 patients followed, who had been assigned to this group for one or multiple reasons. In view of this imbalance between the two prognostic groups, the standards regarding maximum mortality (30 percent as against 62 percent observed deaths) were clearly invalid. The quality assurance coordinator attributed the lack of any subsequent action to effect improvement to the ambivalent attitudes of the staff physicians in this respect. Also, he was concerned by the fact that hardly any patients had received rehabilitative care, such as physical or speech therapy, following discharge, although cooperative arrangements were subsequently made with other clinics for home therapists to follow their stroke patients. This development may or may not have been related to the health accounting project conducted.

The outcome assessment results in the second stroke project (Study 57) indicated little difference overall between findings and standards, yet the staff went ahead with a case-by-case analysis for correctable determinants of what they considered deficient care outcomes. Analysis of the 39 percent death rate yielded inadequate data for a determination of whether these deaths had been preventable.

Table 8.19.   Health care assessment results in four studies of cerebral and cardiovascular disease in adults

Provider Characteristics	Patient and Sample Characteristics	Diagnostic Outcomes[a] (as percent in each category)		Therapeutic Outcomes (as percent at each level)			Sample Size (n) and Completion Rate (percent)			
		Obs	MAS		Obs	MAS	Diagnostic n	%	Therapeutic n	%
Study 9 Facility 3										
University affiliated city hospital in an eastern metropolis. 71 house staff	Working and poverty class adults. Prospective sampling of consecutive coronary care unit admissions of acute myocardial infarction suspects in 6 months; 1 year followup	(n = 75) False negatives[a] 3	5	(n = 75) Asymptomatic, normal and high risk	4	10	122	93	75	100
		(n = 73) False positives[a] 0	5	Symptomatic	35	32				
				Restricted	23	11				
				Dependent	8	17				
				Dead	30	30				
Study 19 Facility 7					Obs	* MAS				
Private fee for service clinic in a suburban eastern town. 20 physicians	Middle and working class adults. Retrospective 1 year sampling of consecutive hospital charts for myocardial infarction suspects followed in referring clinic; 1 year followup			(n = 80) Asymptomatic, normal and high risk	14	23	86		93	
				Symptomatic	9	12				
				Restricted	34	18				
				Dependent	1	16				
				Dead	42	31				

Study 35 Facility 11

Private fee for service clinic in midwest. 29 physicians

Middle and working class adults, mainly > 65 years. Retrospective sampling of hospital charts for consecutive patients with initial cerebrovascular accident (followup period not stated)

	Obs***	MAS	n	%
(n = 86)			100	86
Asymptomatic, normal and high risk	10	1		
Symptomatic	20	10		
Restricted	6	20		
Dependent	2	39		
Dead	62	30		

Study 57 Facility 23

University hospital department of physical medicine and rehabilitation in midwestern metropolis. 31 department physicians

Poverty and working class adults < 60 years. Retrospective sampling of hospital charts for 8 year period for patients with initial cerebrovascular accident; 3–13 year followup

	Obs	+ MAS	n	%
(n = 110)			119	92
Asymptomatic, normal risk	0	0		
Asymptomatic, high risk	3	0		
Symptomatic [b]	9	9		
Restricted [c]	30	20		
Dependent [d]	19	41		
Dead	39	30		

[a] Determined by independent chart review compared with diagnosis of attending physician.

[b] Defined as experiencing reduced comfort and activity (mild) and as requiring some help with self-care (moderate to severe).

[c] Defined as significantly employed but unable to resume full activity (partly restricted) and as active and mainly capable of self-care but not in usual major activity (significantly restricted).

[d] Defined as needing help with self-care and not in usual major activity (partly dependent) and as not capable of self-care or of major activity.

+ $P < 0.1$

* $P < 0.05$

*** $P < 0.001$

Table 8.20.   Therapeutic outcomes in a group of myocardial infarction suspects followed for one year, by prognostic group

	Study 19			
	Prognostic Group			
	Good (n = 36)		Poor (n = 44)	
Therapeutic Outcomes (as percent at each level)	Observed	MAS	Observed	MAS
Asymptomatic, normal and high risk	25	45	5	5
Symptomatic	8	15	9	10
Restricted	36	15	32	20
Dependent	0	10	2	20
Dead	31	15	52	45

Further analysis of a random sample of 50 out of the 110 patients by two independent teams, however, indicated that there was indeed much room for improvement; at least this was concluded for 10 of the 50 patients by Team 1 and for 7 of the 50 by Team 2. Combining these estimates, it is probably safe to say that improvement was judged possible in about 1 of 5 patients studied.

Among the factors that were identified, improved followup care in the form of physical therapy and referral for rehabilitation was the major recommendation, inasmuch as investigation revealed that among the roughly 1 in 5 patients who might have benefited from some form of altered management, two-thirds might have had significantly different health outcomes with this type of care.

Subsequently, the department of physical medicine and rehabilitation of the facility did implement a continuity of care plan (Anderson, 1964). However, at that time, new internal administrative arrangements and external financial arrangements were necessary to implement this plan, since Medicare did not cover such followup. A formal recommendation for national legislative action by a collaborative policy research institute was subsequently formulated for presentation to Congress (Ellwood, 1975). Local action to improve care of these stroke patients was also taken, and new health outcomes were to be evaluated in a subsequent study.

Implications
These four therapeutic outcome assessments have common clinical factors. In each, there seemed to be fewer patients back to their usual

life activities than was considered acceptable. In each, subsequent investigation revealed rather serious neglect of followup care and rehabilitation. In both myocardial infarction studies, the impairment measured could not be attributed to heart pathology. In the two stroke studies, the neglect of posthospital rehabilitation, though confined to a smaller subset, was equally obvious. In three of four instances, action was taken subsequent to the studies to improve followup rehabilitation, and even in Study 35, where the staff had rejected the implications of the findings, a neurologist was added to the clinic staff, and greater emphasis was placed on definitive diagnoses of the causes underlying strokes.

The results suggest that routine vocational evaluation and, if indicated, rehabilitation might be important to all patients discharged alive from hospital care for myocardial infarction, especially those whose diagnosis proved unrelated to heart pathology. Likewise, for stroke patients, followup evaluation and, if indicated, further rehabilitation in relation to motor and speech function would seem essential.

Perhaps the most important ancillary finding in these studies concerned the lack of Medicare financial provisions for followup rehabilitative care. The fact that direct action was taken with regard to policy proposals for further investigation of the problem could have important implications for the health care of such patients in the future.

Quality assurance implications relate to the need for further development of a more sensitive health impairment scale and maximum acceptable health standards. A six level scale was considered inadequate by the study team in Study 57 and was successfully augmented to be more sensitive to the more serious physical impairments of stroke patients. In both Studies 9 and 57, though the maximum acceptable impairment standards were not seriously exceeded, followup study revealed important care deficiencies among small subgroups that might otherwise have been missed.

It was encouraging to note that although one study team denied the significance of the measured deficient findings, they later followed this by taking corrective action. This pattern has been observed in several instances in the health accounting project in different settings and with different problems. It is equally encouraging that by focusing on outcomes, this quality assurance approach can succeed in stimulating inquiry and subsequent action to effect improvement in areas distant from the domain of traditional clinical medicine. That a group of physicians should decide to spend their time and energy on formulating a recommendation for national policy in relation to care cost reimbursement, as happened here, would seem a significant example.

FRACTURES

Topic

A community hospital and a multispecialty clinic selected bone fractures as a study topic, one hospital examining fractures of the lower extremity, mainly tibial, and one clinic Colles' fractures of the distal end of the radius, with or without fracture of the styloid process of the ulna. The providers were orthopedic surgeons in the hospital study and general practitioners and general surgeons in the clinic study. The study population selected by the hospital group consisted of patients discharged after lower leg fractures three years previously and in the clinic of patients having been treated for a wrist fracture at least one year previously. In both studies, the patients were of working and middle class background. Both studies assessed health outcomes.

Design

In both studies, patients were identified retrospectively by searching the file of radiology reports, starting three years prior to the study in the hospital sample and one year prior to the study in the clinic sample and working back in time until approximately 100 consecutive patients had been accumulated in each case. Medical charts were reviewed and a functional impairment questionnaire was mailed out to all patients in the sample. The chart review provided posttreatment x-ray data regarding fracture healing when the cast had been removed and physician evaluation of lower leg or wrist function, deformity, or complications such as infections or arthritis. The followup questionnaire elicited patient assessment of function and cosmetic results with regard to the limb involved. Information was also sought regarding patient satisfaction with the final results of treatment.

Outcome standards in terms of maximum acceptable group impairment not requiring restudy or improvement were set by the staff physicians on the project teams. An extensive literature search was conducted in the hospital study for prognostic data regarding lower leg fractures. In the clinic study of Colles' fractures, three prognostic groups were identified, and separate standards were established for each on the basis of final chart review entries:

- Group 1—No displacement and/or buckle at eight to ten weeks post fracture;
- Group II—Minimal displacement and/or minimum comminution at eight to fourteen weeks post fracture;

Table 8.21. Health care assessment results in two studies of fractures (leg and Colles') in adults

Provider Characteristics	Patient and Sample Characteristics	Therapeutic Outcomes[a] (as percent at each level)	Obs	MAS	Sample Size (n) and Completion Rate (percent) MAS n	%
Study 4 Facility 1						
Community fee for service hospital in midwestern city. 114 physicians	Working and middle class adults. Retrospective sampling of consecutive posttreatment radiology reports (3 years) for lower leg fractures; 3 year posttreatment followup	*Chart Review* (n = 88)			100	88
		Non or malunion	6	5		
		Needs care after 15 months	17	15		
		Limited motion	24	20		
		Complications	4	6.5		
		Patient Questionnaire (n = 44)			88	50
		Impaired running	38	38		
		Impaired walking	18	20		
		Impaired climbing	12	13		
		Visible deformity	37 ***	8		
Study 31 Facility 10			Obs	MAS	MAS n	%
Multispecialty fee for service group clinic in a rural midwestern town. 16 physicians	Working and middle class adults. Retrospective sampling of consecutive posttreatment radiology reports (1 year) for Colles' fractures; 1–3 year posttreatment followup	*Chart Review* (n = 107)	Lack of full function		107	100
		Prognostic Displacement/ Group Comminution				
		I None n = 58	2	0		
		II Moderate n = 44	16	18		
		III Maximal n = 5	0	28		
		Patient Questionnaire (n = 47)			47	44
		Any impairment of wrist	10	19		

[a]Health problem outcomes, measured as complications and functional outcomes. Overall health status not assessed.

***P < 0.001

- Group III—Maximal displacement and/or maximal comminution at twelve to eighteen weeks post fracture.

Results

In Study 4, 88 hospital charts were located for the 100 patients in the sample with a previous lower leg fracture. Chart review revealed all findings to be within maximum acceptable impairment standards, with one in four having limited motion according to the physician notes. This result was not significantly different from the 20 percent standard. Less than one in twenty had a mal- or nonunion, again within standards, as shown in Table 8.21.

Only 44 of the 88 patients contacted by mail completed and returned the health status questionnaire, for a 50 percent response rate. Thirty-seven percent reported a visible deformity of the leg due to the injury, an outcome significantly exceeding standards. A similar proportion in this three year followup study reported impaired ability to run, although this result was within standards considered acceptable.

In Study 31, health outcomes were likewise found to be within acceptable standards for all three prognostic groups. Outcomes at the time of cast removal were studied and compared to the standards established (see Table 8.21). Replies to the one to three year followup questionnaire were obtained for only 47 of the 107 patients, for a 44 percent completion rate. In the group responding, only 10 percent did not report full functional return, a percentage well within standards. Specific functional limitations for this group of Colles' fracture patients are shown in Table 8.22.

Implications

On the face of it, these studies would indicate that the staff have little to learn clinically in these instances, as performance seemed well within their own standards. In the hospital study, where the standards incorporated results of a literature review on prognosis, these standards proved to be credible, in contrast to those set by the clinic staff, where some controversy later arose. The implications of the assessment findings in both studies proved acceptable to the staffs; both groups concluded that no further evaluation of care for patients with these fractures was indicated and that no improvement action was required.

Quality assurance implications, on the other hand, are mixed. In terms of selecting a high priority topic with potential for appreciable patient health improvement, the teams failed if the study results can

Table 8.22. Specific functional limitations in a group of forty-seven Colles' fracture patients one to three years post treatment[a]

		Study 31		
Number of Patients	*Age*	*Sex*	*Pain*	*Limitation*
1	78	F	No	Weak shoulder
1	79	F	No	Cannot fasten brassiere
1	49	F	Yes	Pain on motion of wrist
1	52	F	Yes	Cannot carry heavy objects
1	68	F	No	Severe loss of motion

[a]No symptoms in forty-two patients.

be considered valid. In the clinic study, it was revealed later that there was a conscious effort to preclude choice of a topic that would make the clinic look bad. The staff seemed quite sensitive to the possibility of adverse publicity in a small town. The same clinic would later drop out of the health accounting program.

However, the major weakness in both studies was that the response rates for the questionnaire were only 50 and 44 percent, respectively. The patients not responding may have had seriously deficient results; they may have gone to other physicians or have been so dissatisfied that they were not willing to cooperate in the study. On the other hand, the nonrespondents may indeed have been similar to the respondents. Whichever was the case, it is not possible to determine the overall validity of the results based on the data provided or to generalize them to the total group of patients.

REFERENCES

Anderson, E.M. 1964. A continuity-of-care plan for long-term patients. *Am J Pub Health* 54:308–12.

Cahill, G.F., Jr.; Ertzwiler, L.D.; and Freinkel, N. 1976. "Control" and diabetes. *N Engl J Med* 294:1004–05, 1029.

Dershewitz, R. 1977. Personal communication.

———. 1975. Urinary tract infection—prevention, recurrence and significance. Conclusions from the literature. Baltimore: Johns Hopkins School of Hygiene and Public Health (processed).

Ellwood, P. 1975. Personal communication.

Goldner, M.G.; Knatterud, G.L.; and Prout, T.E. 1971. Effects of hypoglycemic agents in vascular complications in patients with adult onset diabetes, pt. 3: Clinical complications of UGDP results. *JAMA* 218:1400–10.

Medical Letter. 1974. Microstix and other office tests for the detection of urinary tract infection. *Medical Letter* 16(3) Issue 393:13–15.

University Group Diabetes Program. 1970. A study of the effects of hypo-glycemic agents on vascular complications in patients with adult-onset diabetes, pt. 1: Design, methods and baseline results; pt. 2: Mortality results. *Diabetes* 19(suppl. 2):747–85, 787–830.

Chapter 9

Health Accounting Outcome Studies: Surgery, Laboratory Procedures, and Prenatal Screening

This chapter will focus on a set of therapeutic outcomes for patients categorized by specific management interventions such as surgical procedures and screening tests, and on diagnostic outcomes in a series of laboratory procedure studies where outcomes were assessed in terms of adequate physician response to abnormal test results.

SURGICAL OPERATIONS

Four clinics and their associated hospitals elected to study outcomes for patients receiving surgical operations. Five categories of surgical procedures were studied: cholecystectomy, hemorrhoidectomy, cataractectomy, hysterectomy, and endarterectomy. The outcome emphasis in these studies was on both overall health status and specific health problem status.

Cholecystectomy

Topic. In two studies of cholecystectomy selected for quality assurance, most of the providers were board certified surgeons. The patient groups were mainly of working class background, with some middle class patients in Study 2, and they were seen on a fee for service basis. All had undergone a cholecystectomy. The health outcomes studied were related to health problem status in terms of patient function and complications of the operative procedure.

Design. Study 2 involved a retrospective sample of approximately 300 consecutive patients who had undergone cholecystectomy five or more years previously; in Study 24, retrospective sampling extended to all patients operated on during an eighteen-month period, for an average of one year prior to the investigation. The sample comprised 222 patients.

A chart review and followup encounter form were developed, although the chart review form was not available in time for Study 2. In Study 24, this form included patient identification, dates of hospital admission, operation, and discharge; operative notes regarding common duct explorations or T-tube use; and complications during or immediately after surgery. The followup questionnaire in both studies covered questions regarding symptoms related to the operation, its complications, and subsequent gastrointestinal symptoms, and in Study 24 several questions related to satisfaction with care received.

In Study 2, the followup encounter form was mailed to patients; and in Study 24, a telephone survey was conducted, followed by mailouts to those not available by telephone. Assessment standards were set by team consensus, supported by a limited literature review.

Results. For the 300 patient sample in Study 2, replies were received from 193, for a 64 percent response rate. In Study 24, 218 patients were contacted out of the 222 patient sample, for a 98 percent response rate (Table 9.1).

The findings did not conform to maximum acceptable impairment standards in either study. Study 2 identified more patients than acceptable by agreed standards as symptomatic or restricted in their activities, 9 percent having required additional surgery for the problem. In both studies, the significant impairment identified related primarily to the inordinate number of patients reporting the same symptoms experienced prior to surgery at the time of interview. Abdominal pain and fatty food intolerance were the main symptoms recorded in both studies. In Study 2, seven patients reported postsurgical jaundice as well. In Study 24, the surgeons reviewed the findings on the symptomatic patients and concluded that most of the symptoms were probably unrelated to the surgery; they also found that common duct exploration did not seem to have had any effect in terms of outcomes measured. In terms of patient satisfaction, 87 percent of the 218 patients responding in Study 24 rated their care as excellent and 10 percent as good.

Implications. The clinical implications of these studies are open to question. Aside from the limited review by the physicians in

Table 9.1. Health care assessment results in two studies of cholecystectomies in adults

Provider Characteristics	Patient and Sample Characteristics	Therapeutic Outcomes (as percent at each level)		Sample Size (n) and Completion Rate (percent)	
		Obs***	MAS	n	%
Study 2 Facility 1					
Community hospital and fee for service clinic in midwestern city. 114 physicians	Working and some middle class adults. Retrospective sampling of consecutive hospital charts for cholecystectomies; 5 year followup	(n = 193) Asymptomatic, normal and high risk		300	64
		50	85		
		Symptomatic 37	12		
		Restricted[a] 9	3		
		Dependent 0	0		
		Dead 4	0		
		Obs**	MAS	n	%
Study 24 Facility 9					
Fee for service clinic and hospital in midwestern town. 115 physicians	Working class adults. Retrospective sampling of consecutive hospital charts (18 months) for cholecystectomies; 1 year average followup	(n = 218) Asymptomatic, normal and high risk		222	98
		64.5	75		
		Symptomatic 31	13		
		Restricted 3	6		
		Dependent 1	3		
		Dead 0.5	3		

[a]Defined as reoperated for biliary tract disease.

Note: In Tables 9.1–9.17, the abbreviations Obs and MAS denote, respectively, observed results and maximum acceptable standards. See Chapter 7 for methods used to determine statistical significance.

**P < 0.01

***P < 0.001

Study 24, no systematic effort was made to evaluate symptomatic patients, despite the fact that the number of patients who were re-operated and who reported jaundice and abdominal pain should have been sufficient evidence to suggest a followup clinical study of chole-cystectomy patients. A more extensive literature review to establish the efficacy of treatment would appear to be the least effort that should have been made in the circumstances.

Quality assurance implications are equally discouraging. The study teams had set standards indicating that more than 15 or 25 percent, respectively, of symptomatic, otherwise restricted, or dead patients would be considered unacceptable. Observed findings were 50 percent and 35 percent, respectively. Since the study teams, at least in Study 24, were not too concerned about the findings, they would have to admit that their prognostic judgment as encompassed in the standards was questionable. In the absence of further evidence from the literature or of an in-depth followup of the patients involved, one would be hesitant to give accolades for quality, whether of the clinical results in terms of outcomes measured or of the general assessment effort.

Hemorrhoidectomy

Topic. In a hemorrhoidectomy quality assurance study conducted by one clinic and hospital, the providers were board certified surgeons, one a specialist in proctology. The patients were primarily of working class background, with some middle class patients included. Therapeutic outcomes were primarily assessed in terms of patient function, symptoms, and satisfaction.

Design. The retrospective consecutive sample consisted of 400 patients having received a hemorrhoidectomy at least two years prior to the investigation. A mailout questionnaire was developed to elicit information on symptoms, signs, patient function, and satisfaction with results; this being one of the earliest health accounting studies, the overall health scale used in most subsequent studies was not yet available. Standards were set by team consensus and subsequently confirmed by a literature review.

Results. Of the 400 questionnaires mailed out, response was obtained from only 204, yielding a 51 percent response rate. An average interval of three years had passed since the hemorrrhoidectomy for those who did respond.

The findings were mixed (Table 9.2). A greater than acceptable

Table 9.2.   Health care assessment results in a study of hemorrhoidectomies in adults

Provider Characteristics	Patient and Sample Characteristics	Therapeutic Outcomes[a] (as percent at each level)			Sample Size (n) and Completion Rate (percent)	
			Obs	MAS	n	%
Study 5 Facility 1						
Community hospital and fee for service clinic in midwestern city. 114 physicians	Working and some middle class adults. Retrospective sampling of hospital charts for consecutive hemorrhoidectomies dating back 2 years or more; 3 year average followup	*Postsurgery Function*			400	51
		(n = 202)				
		Poor bowel control	30***12			
		(n = 199)				
		Abnormal bowel movements	14	20		
		(n = 204)				
		Small stools	22 **12			
		(n = 187)				
		Work absence >4 weeks	16	15		
		Postsurgery Symptoms				
		(n = 204)				
		Rectal discomfort	13 +	10		
		Rectal bleeding	11 +	7		
		Rectal protrusion	10	12		

[a]Health problem outcomes in terms of postsurgery function and symptoms for specific problem; overall health status not assessed.

+P < 0.1
**P < 0.01
***P < 0.001

proportion of patients reported poor bowel control, abnormally small stools, and rectal bleeding and discomfort, although the proportion of patients with abnormal bowel movements, excessive absence from work, and rectal protrusion was within acceptable limits. However, the literature review conducted independently of team standard-setting procedures provided remarkably similar findings.

Only 13 percent of the respondents expressed dissatisfaction with surgical results or were reluctant to recommend the procedure to others. This compares favorably with the team's maximum acceptable dissatisfaction standard, which had been set at 15 percent.

Implications. The clinical implications of this evaluation are open to several questions. The fact that both team standards and literature findings were exceeded by a factor of two in regard to poor bowel control several years after surgery seems worthy of attention. The deficiencies in relation to postsurgery symptoms such as small stools, rectal discomfort, and rectal bleeding were not substantial, although the difference from standards was significant at the $P < 0.1$ level. The fact that the investigating team took no further action may be implicit confirmation that they really were not too disturbed by the deficiencies found.

Quality assurance implications relate to the sampling and survey methods applied. The most serious drawback here was the low response rate (51 percent), which probably precludes generalization to the universe of hemorrhoidectomy patients managed by these surgeons. The standards seemed realistic, the efficacy of the procedure in question being documented by the team's literature search. The high patient satisfaction rate is difficult to evaluate.

Hysterectomy

Topic. One rural multispecialty clinic and associated hospital elected to study hysterectomies. The physicians were either board eligible or board certified in obstetrics and gynecology; patients were working class women from a surrounding rural population who had undergone a hysterectomy within a two year period. Outcomes in terms of overall patient health status and function were assessed.

Design. A retrospective, consecutive one in two sampling of all patients receiving either a vaginal or abdominal hysterectomy in a two year period yielded a sample of 297 patients. The sample frame

Table 9.3.   Health care assessment results in a study of hysterectomies

Provider Characteristics	Patient and Sample Characteristics	Therapeutic Outcomes (as percent at each level)		Sample Size (n) and Completion Rate (percent)	
		Obs	MAS	n	%
Study 28 Facility 9					
Fee for service clinic and hospital in a midwestern town. 115 physicians	Working class adult females. Retrospective one in two sampling of surgery register for consecutive vaginal or abdominal hysterectomies in 2 year period; 1 year average followup	(n = 276) Asymptomatic, normal and high risk		297	93
		high risk	64	50	
		Symptomatic	30	40	
		Restricted	4	7	
		Dependent	0.5	1	
		Dead	1.5	2	

consisted of the surgery register of all operations performed in the hospital.

Outcome measures were obtained by patient questionnaires administered by telephone and by a chart review form. The hospital charts were reviewed to identify recorded diagnoses; date of admission, operation, and discharge for the hysterectomy; and any complications related to the operative procedure. Patients were classified according to vaginal and abdominal hysterectomies and were asked the standard questions underlying the six level health scale (see Chapter 6) to determine their level of health and function. A mailout questionnaire was used when no telephone contact was possible. Assessment standards were established by team consensus in terms of the maximum acceptable disability of the total sample, with the first and second levels of the six level scale collapsed.

Results. Of the 297 patients sampled, results were obtained from 276, yielding an overall response rate of 93 percent. Of 89 patients with a vaginal hysterectomy, 88 responded; of the 208 with an abdominal hysterectomy, 188 responded.

As shown in Table 9.3, observed outcomes were well within the standards set by the team. There was no appreciable difference in outcomes for the 88 respondents who had received a vaginal hysterectomy as compared to the 188 who underwent abdominal hysterectomy.

Implications. On the face of it, the clinical implications of this study indicate that adequate care was provided by the physicians involved. However, it appears that the bare minimum of adequate information was obtained. There is no mention of any literature review supporting team assessment standards nor any mention of indications for hysterectomies or of complication rates; assessment standards and measures in this respect would clearly have provided important information to support the validity of the findings. Also, the fact that no improvement potential was identified raises questions regarding the judgment applied in selecting this topic in the first place.

Cataractectomy

Topic. One clinic elected to assess outcomes for patients who had operations for cataracts by three board certified ophthalmologists. The patients were mainly elderly (average age, 71.4 years), retired working and middle class males and females, half from the surrounding rural farm area and local towns and half from the city where the clinic was located. Outcomes were assessed both in terms of overall patient health and functioning and of specific measures of postoperative visual acuity.

Design. A retrospective consecutive sample of all patients who underwent cataractectomy during a one year period was drawn. The sample frame consisted of a computerized patient record system in the hospital where the operations were performed, and the sample was restricted to patients of the ophthalmologists in the clinic participating in the study, yielding 113 patients.

The assessment measure consisted of a patient questionnaire administered by telephone interview and a chart review form. The patient questionnaire elicited answers to the standard questions underlying assignment of each patient to one level on the six level health scale (see Chapter 6). The chart review form used to record data from both hospital and clinic records covered dates of hospitalization, including the date of the operative procedure, history of any previous eye surgery, all diagnoses indicating systemic as well as ocular disease, family history of ocular disease, and information regarding patient compliance, as well as all visual acuity data.

For health problem outcome assessment, patients were classified into two prognostic groups based on the following:

	Weights
Age (<40 or >79)	1
Drugs (Indocin, steroids, chlorpromazine, thorazine, or folic acid antagonists)	1
Welfare support	1
Family history of ocular disease	2
Noncompliance (does not follow directions or accept ophthalmic correction)	3
Related systemic disease	4
Previous ocular surgery	4
Other ocular disease	4

Patients were assigned to the worst prognostic group if they had six or more points. Health problem outcome standards were established by consensual judgment of the project study team, with little or no formal literature search conducted to support standards.

Results. The overall response rate was 94 percent. The assessment findings for both health problem and overall health and disability outcomes are shown in Table 9.4. The results for both visual acuity

Table 9.4.   Health care assessment results in a study of cataractectomies in elderly adults

Provider Characteristics	Patient and Sample Characteristics	Therapeutic Outcomes[a] (as percent at each level)				Sample Size (n) and Completion Rate (percent)	
			Obs	MAS	Obs	MAS	n	%
Study 11 Facility 4								
Fee for service clinic and hospital in midwestern rural town. 26 physicians	Working and middle class elderly adults (average age 71.4 years). Retrospective sampling of patient records for consecutive cataractectomies performed by participating ophthalmologists; 1 year followup	Better Prognostic Group (n = 40) Visual acuity			(n = 106) Asymptomatic, normal and high risk	61	29	113	94
		20/20–20/40	92	78	Symptomatic	14	30	
		20/50–20/200	8	16	Restricted	8	21	
		<20/200	0	6	Dependent	6	15	
		Worst Prognostic Group (n = 66) Visual acuity			Dead	11	5	
		20/20–20/40	75	52				
		20/50–20/200	21	27				
		<20/200	4	21				

[a]Including visual acuity outcomes by prognostic group.

and overall health status were much more favorable than anticipated, except for a higher than anticipated proportion of deaths. In terms of visual acuity, the worst prognostic group showed a corresponding outcome. Systemic disease was the major contributor to the number of prognostic points accrued, but even here, the results were within standards.

An interesting relationship noted was the fact that patients who subjectively felt that their vision was not as good as they expected also had difficulty accepting ophthalmic correction and had to be seen more often to complete their care. The converse was also marked, in that those pleased with the results also accepted correction and were seen much less frequently to complete care. However, objectively measured postoperative visual acuity was within standards for both groups.

Implications. This study indicates that performance in this area did not require improvement action at the time. Outcomes were within acceptable standards, and the apparent validity of the prognostic scale was a valuable finding. The ophthalmologists involved stated that they would be hesitant to operate on future patients having a high score.

On the other hand, despite the high response rate obtained, the lack of any literature review to support the validity of the outcome assessment standards leaves some question as to the significance of the measured findings. The coordinator in this clinic also noted an evident bias in selecting the topic, the staff being anxious to study an area where they were likely to excel. While this was a common tendency in initial health accounting projects, such attitudes lead to a wasteful use of quality assurance effort, the main purpose of which is to establish improvement potential.

Carotid Endarterectomy

Topic. One clinic and associated hospital investigated carotid endarterectomy as a quality assurance topic. The providers were mostly board certified surgeons, including a vascular surgical specialist, and internists and radiologists on the staff of the clinic and the affiliated hospital. The patient group consisted largely of working class individuals from a mixed industrial-mining-farming area in the south central United States. Therapeutic outcomes were assessed in terms of overall health status of endarterectomy patients.

Design. A retrospective consecutive sample of approximately 100 patients who had undergone this operation during a four year period was drawn from the surgery register for the hospital where the operations had been performed. The standard patient health status questionnaire for evaluating overall functional disability was applied by telephone interview or by personal interview at the hospital or in the patient's home if telephone contact was not feasible. In addition, a chart review was completed for each patient regarding age, dates of hospitalization and surgery, serious associated systemic disease, coronary heart disease, and symptoms, signs, and laboratory work related to carotid and intracerebral artery disease.

Patients were assigned to three prognostic groups, the best prognostic group including those of all ages without serious associated systemic disease (diabetes mellitus, hypertension in excess of 100 diastolic blood pressure, or lipid abnormalities) and those with such associated disease but under age 60. The intermediate prognostic group consisted of patients over 60 with associated systemic disease (diabetes mellitus, hypertension, and/or lipid abnormalities); and the worst prognostic group, of patients with coronary artery disease (EKG abnormalities, documented myocardial infarction, and/or angina pectoris). Assessment standards indicating maximum acceptable group disability were established by team consensus.

Results.   Of a total sample of 112 consecutive patients with an endarterectomy in the four year sampling period, complete data were obtained from 104, for a 93 percent response rate. Table 9.5 shows that in terms of overall therapeutic outcomes, results fell short of maximum acceptable standards for the group as a whole; this was true also for each of three prognostic subgroups (Table 9.6).

The major factor seemed to be the high number of deaths, the observed rate being nearly three times the maximum acceptable rate. The proportion of patients who had not returned to major life activity or were dependent was likewise high, and similar relationships held for all three prognostic groups. Table 9.7 shows the distribution among the prognostic groups of clinical characteristics of the 104 patients studied, and Table 9.8 indicates additional data obtained from chart review on those who had died within the followup period. Available data regarding the cause of death and/or occurrence of strokes were considered inadequate in 15 cases. It should be noted that the physicians themselves had attempted to follow these patients by written requests for a return visit, but only eight patients finally returned.

Implications.   The clinical implications of these findings are sobering. Some 60 percent of 104 patients were unable to return to their

Table 9.5. Health care assessment results in a study of carotid endarterectomies in adults

Provider Characteristics	Patient and Sample Characteristics	Therapeutic Outcomes (as percent at each level)		Sample Size (n) and Completion Rate (percent)	
		Obs***	MAS	n	%
Study 38 Facility 13					
Fee for service clinic and hospital in south central rural town. 50 physicians	Working class adults. Retrospective sampling of surgery register for consecutive carotid endarterectomies in 4 year period; average postoperative followup 1.5 years	(n = 104)		112	93
		Asymptomatic, normal and high risk 12	37		
		Symptomatic 26	29		
		Restricted 29	17		
		Dependent 7	8		
		Dead 26	9		

***P < 0.001

Table 9.6. Therapeutic outcomes for a group of carotid endarterectomy patients followed for one to three years, by prognostic group

	Study 38					
	Prognostic Group					
Therapeutic Outcomes (as percent at each level)	Best[a] (n = 31)		Intermediate[b] (n = 16)		Worst[c] (n = 57)	
	Obs	MAS	Obs	MAS	Obs	MAS
Asymptomatic, normal and high risk	23	45	6	42	7	32
Symptomatic	19	31	50	29	23	27
Restricted	26	15	19	15	35	19
Dependent	6	4	6	7	7	10
Dead	26	5	19	7	28	12

[a]No associated systemic disease *or* associated systemic disease, but under age sixty.
[b]Over age sixty with associated systemic disease.
[c]With coronary artery disease.

Table 9.7. Distribution of clinical characteristics in 104 carotid endarterectomy patients, by prognostic group

		Study 38			
			Prognostic Group		
	Clinical Characteristics	All Patients	Best	Intermediate	Worst
Age	<60	15	8	0	7
	>60	89	23	16	50
Symptoms	Transient ischemic attacks	83	25	12	46
	Bruits	85	25	13	47
	Petite stroke	49	13	9	27
	Ophthalmological findings	23	6	2	15
Systemic Disease	Diabetes mellitus	9	0	4	5
	Hypertension[a]	20	4	11	5
	Lipid abnormalities	6	0	3	3
	Coronary artery disease	18	0	0	18
	EKG abnormalities	48	0	0	48
	Documented myocardial infarction	19	0	0	19
	Angina pectoris	16	0	0	16

[a]In excess of 100 diastolic blood pressure.

Table 9.8.   Data on twenty-four deaths after carotid endarterectomy[a]

	Study 38
Item	*Number of Cases*
Chart review completed	23
Average survival time following surgery	11 months 22 days
Number autopsied	4
Cause of death	
Cerebrovascular accident	5
Myocardial infarction	12
Uremia	2
Cancer	2
Ruptured aortic aneurysm	1
Mesenteric artery thrombosis	1
Cerebrovascular accident symptoms before death	13
Cerebrovascular accident after surgery	8
No postoperative care recorded[b]	15

[a]Obtained from chart review.
[b]Letter requesting followup visit written in all fifteen cases; eight complied.

major life activity, bedridden, or dead at an average of eighteen months post surgery. These findings far exceeded acceptable impairment standards set by the surgical staff on the basis of their knowledge and experience with these patients, who were recognized as being a very high risk group. Serious questions arise as to the accuracy of the preoperative diagnoses, indications for applying this operative procedure, and possible problems in operative technique and followup care provided. The fact that the observed death and disability rates did not vary markedly among prognostic groupings would seem significant. The criteria and standards applied by the staff would certainly indicate reinvestigation, and an in-depth literature review would probably have provided helpful data for this purpose. The quality assurance coordinator stated that subsequent record review had indicated no appreciable mortality or morbidity from the diagnostic procedure (carotid arteriogram) or the surgery (carotid endarterectomy). One wonders whether and to what extent this conclusion was self-serving, especially in view of the fact that carotid arteriograms are high risk procedures with significant morbidity even in the best of cases.

The quality assurance implications of this study are equally significant. The physicians on the study team were "happy" with the health outcome standards they had developed immediately after the study design meeting. After seeing the results, however, the group expressed serious doubts regarding these standards. At a subsequent meeting they attempted to derive more valid standards but failed because they felt that the patients had so many other complicating conditions. On the other hand, the group reexamined the measured findings and concluded that they were accurate. Overall, these surgeons rejected the study on the basis that they had tried to evaluate whether or not strokes were being prevented by this operative procedure and that the study failed to yield such information.

This finding is most important in that it emphasizes the fact that quality assurance assessment studies cannot establish, but at best provide clues for, the efficacy of clinical interventions. In general, assessment studies should not be designed if efficacy of clinical management is not accepted from the outset and, if possible, documented.

Followup personal communications with the quality assurance coordinator did lead to a surprising observation, however. Although the surgeons on the study team did not admit that performance deficiencies had been identified by this study, their subsequent practice behavior did seem to change. It was observed that they became much more stringent in their indications for surgery. In the coordinator's opinion, the number of such operations was in fact reduced subsequent to the assessment study. This is an interesting example that is quite the opposite of the frequent admission of deficient performance by staff who then do nothing about it (Williamson, Alexander, and Miller, 1967). The coordinator further attested that this study had important educational value in terms of staff understanding of the natural history of patients with carotid artery occlusive disease.

LABORATORY TESTS

A similar group of clinics and/or their affiliated hospitals elected to study outcomes with regard to physician response to screening laboratory tests. Six different test procedures were studied: hemoglobin tests, hematocrits, fasting blood sugars, urinalyses, electrocardiograms, and intravenous pyelograms.

In these studies, manifest physician responses to reported test abnormalities were defined as the outcome to be measured. If this outcome did not meet specified standards, detailed inquiry into related processes was considered indicated. The studies described in the following represent a typical outcome assessment in the area of diagnostic management.

Hemoglobin and Hematrocrit Tests

Topic. Two clinics studied the results of physicians ordering hemoglobin or hematocrit tests on their patients. The providers were the total staff of a community hospital in Study 1c and a large multi-specialty group practice in Study 27. The patients in both studies were predominantly of working class background, with some middle class patients, from a small city and a rural town in the Midwest. Diagnostic outcomes were evaluated in terms of physician response to reported unexpected abnormal test results.

Design. A retrospective random sample of blood hemoglobin test results (Study 1c) and a retrospective consecutive sample of hemato-crits (Study 27) were studied to determine unexpected abnormalities, that is, abnormal test results not related to the admitting diagnosis. The sample frame in both cases was the laboratory file of duplicate test report slips.

The assessment measure in both studies consisted of a chart review to determine whether the physician had made an appropriate response to the unexpected test result, defined as (1) a repeat test to confirm the abnormality, or (2) any effort to identify the etiology of the abnormal result if treatment was given. Abnormal results were defined as follows:

Hemoglobin	*Hematocrit*
≥33 percent below normal value for age	Male ≤39.9%
Adults: Male ≤11gm/100cc	Female ≤34.9%
Female ≤10 gm/100cc	
Children: Adjusted for age	
(Karger, 1959)	

In both clinics, the staff considered that every abnormal test result should receive an appropriate response as defined above, so that the maximum acceptable standard for nonresponses was zero.

In Study 1c, a table of random numbers was used to select a sample of hemoglobin tests reported for each of five nonconsecutive months six months apart. In Study 27, a retrospective consecutive sample of 100 abnormal hematocrit values was obtained from a total of 888 laboratory test reports.

Results. As shown in Table 9.9, standards were not met in either study. In Study 1c, the validity of the observed substantial perfor-

Table 9.9.   Health care assessment results in two studies of abnormal hemoglobin and hematocrit tests

Provider Characteristics	Patient and Sample Characteristics	Diagnostic Outcomes[a] (as percent in each category)				Sample Size (n) and Completion Rate (percent)	
		Obs	MAS	n		n	%
Study 1c Facility 1							
Community hospital in a midwestern city. 114 physicians	Working and some middle class patients. Retrospective random sampling of laboratory duplicate test report file for 5 nonconsecutive months for unexpected abnormal hemoglobin test results[b]	(n = 32) Lack of minimum adequate response	84 ***	0		32	100
Study 27 Facility 9		Obs	MAS				
Rural clinic in a midwestern town. 115 physicians	Working class patients. Retrospective consecutive sampling of hematocrit test reports for abnormal results[c]	(n = 100) Lack of minimum adequate response	14 ***	0		888	100

[a]Diagnostic outcomes measured in terms of physician response to abnormal test results.
[b]$\leqslant$33 percent of normal value for age.
[c]$\leqslant$39.9% for males, $\leqslant$34.9% for females.
***P < 0.001

mance deficiency (84 percent as compared to a standard of 0 percent) was confirmed by the study team through followup chart review of both hospital and clinic charts for each patient. The physicians also reviewed a sample of their own charts for evidence of any circumstances that could explain the deficiency. The physicians agreed that the deficient results were serious in terms of risk to patient health; following detailed inquiry, they acknowledged that they were personally responsible for the deficient outcomes.

In Study 27, the response to test abnormalities in 14 percent of the sample was likewise judged deficient on first screening. Further investigation of the charts convinced these physicians, however, that all patients had received satisfactory medical care. The only admitted deficiency related to inadequacy of followup notes in the charts, but not to the care provided.

Implications. The clinical implications of these early studies are mixed. In Study 1c, the observed deficiencies were considered to be a serious risk to patient health. While subsequent studies regarding the prognosis for hemoglobin levels between 10 and 13 gm/100cc have raised questions as to the significance of such findings (McKeown, 1968), few would deny that findings below 10 gm/100cc are potentially serious. Consequently, to correct deficiencies in such instances, it would seem important at least to verify observed abnormalities and to identify their causes.

In Study 27, the clinical significance of hematocrits between 30 and 40 percent may be open to question. However, if such a definition of abnormality is indeed questionable, the finding of adequate physician response in this study (86 percent), if interpreted as treatment of all such patients, would raise questions as to an overdiagnosis of anemia. Unfortunately, neither the frequency distribution of the abnormalities nor the relation of adequate response to treatment prescribed was reported by the study team so that further assessment must remain speculative.

On the other hand, the quality assurance implications in these studies are of interest. The hematocrit study in particular illustrates the importance of adequately documenting the efficacy of health care prior to designing an assessment study. If a review of controlled trials indicates that treatment of mild iron deficiency anemia makes little difference to patient health, such patients might well be excluded from study. Likewise, if the team judgment is that present care is probably effective, then further study might be questionable. In health accounting, a consensus of knowledgeable staff on the likelihood of effecting health improvement is required before such a study is designed. If a high proportion of completed studies determine that the outcomes and processes of care in a particular content area are adequate, then extensive further effort would seem wasted. The validity of team projections regarding potential for health impact remains to be conclusively demonstrated, although initial evidence is now available supporting it (Williamson et al., 1977).

Fasting Blood Sugar

Topic.   In a related study, the providers were again the physician staff of a community hospital in a midwestern city. Most patients were from middle and working class backgrounds. The outcome topic was adequacy of physician response to serious unexpected blood sugar test abnormalities found in routine screening for fasting blood sugar.

Design.   A retrospective random sample of screening fasting blood sugar (FBS) laboratory test reports indicating serious abnormality unrelated to the admitting diagnosis was drawn from the pool of all FBS tests run during each of five nonconsecutive months six months apart. Serious abnormality was interpreted as 130 mg% or more of glucose.

The charts for each patient included in the sample were reviewed to determine whether the responsible physician had provided minimum adequate response, which in this case was a repeat test consisting of a two hour postprandial blood sugar, or any explicit evidence that the abnormality was communicated to the referring physician, if applicable.

Standards were again set at 0 percent; in other words, the staff would not accept any instances of over 130 mg% of glucose to go unheeded.

Results.   A total of 63 unexpected abnormal fasting blood sugar laboratory reports were included in the random sample. A chart review was completed for each of the respective medical records containing the laboratory report. The results, as shown in Table 9.10, revealed that 68 percent of reported abnormalities in screening fasting blood sugar tests failed to elicit adequate or appropriate physician response. The physicians did not subsequently establish definitive diagnoses or confirm the abnormal results reported; in most instances, the records did not even indicate that they were in any way aware of the abnormal results of the laboratory report.

Table 9.10. Health care assessment results in a study of elevated fasting blood sugar levels

Provider Characteristics	Patient and Sample Characteristics	Diagnostic Outcomes[a] (as percent in each category)		Sample Size (n) and Completion Rate (percent)	
		Obs	MAS	n	%
Study 1b Facility 1					
Community hospital in a midwestern city. 114 physicians	Working and some middle class patients. Retrospective random sampling of laboratory test report file for 5 nonconsecutive months for unexpected abnormal screening fasting blood sugar test results[b]	(n = 63) Lack of minimum adequate response 68 ***	0	63	100

[a]Diagnostic outcomes measured in terms of physician response to abnormal test results.
[b]≥ 130 mg% glucose.
***P < 0.001

Implications. The clinical implications of this study may have become somewhat controversial since the results of the University Group Diabetes Program (1970) raised questions regarding the value of identifying asymptomatic, insulin independent diabetes such as that constituted by glucose tolerance abnormalities. Many of the subjects in this study probably fitted this category. Aside from this consideration, however, the lack of adequate response in 68 percent of reported cases of unexpected FBS in excess of 130 mg% would seem a serious deficiency in physician performance. As a minimum, a check to determine how many of these in fact represented uncontrolled insulin dependent diabetes would have appeared advisable.

The quality assurance implications of this study confirm the value of an initial outcome screening study. A potentially serious deficiency was uncovered, and specific directions for subsequent inquiry were identified. Inquiry as to why these serious abnormalities were neglected did result. Clinic records for each patient were reviewed and the physicians interviewed. However, the only explanation that was furnished in the study was that the physicians in each case were so preoccupied with other, immediate patient problems that abnormal results of routine screening tests not ordered by the physicians themselves went unnoticed.

Urinalysis

Topic. The same facility that conducted the hemoglobin and FBS studies elected to study physician response to abnormal results of screening urinalyses for consecutive admissions to a community hospital in a midwestern city. The providers were the hospital physician staff responsible for the care of these patients, who were from middle and working class backgrounds. The focus of assessment was again the adequacy of physician response to serious test abnormalities.

Design. A retrospective random sample of screening urinalysis laboratory test reports indicating serious unexpected abnormalities—i.e., unrelated to the admitting diagnosis—was drawn from the pool of all urinalyses run during each of five nonconsecutive months six months apart. Significant abnormalities were interpreted as proteinuria ($\geqslant 1+$) and/or pyuria or hematuria ($\geqslant 5$ white or red blood cells per high power field).

The assessment measure was a chart review of each medical record in the sample to determine whether a minimum adequate response to the abnormal test result had been elicited from the physician, in this case, a repeat urinalysis if proteinuria was recorded; a specific test for bacteriuria if abnormal sediment was noted; or any communication of the abnormal result to the referring physician, if applicable. In this study, standards were again set at 0 percent; in other words, any results below minimum adequate response as defined would be unacceptable.

Results. A total of 164 unexpected abnormal screening urinalysis reports constituted the sample. A chart review was completed in each instance. The results are shown in Table 9.11. Again, in 83 percent of the cases, there was little or no indication that the physician was even aware of the abnormality reported, let alone any indication of repeat tests to confirm the finding or of followup study to determine a definitive diagnosis.

Implications. The clinical implications of this study, too, may be open to question due to the present controversy regarding the benefit of treating asymptomatic bacteriuria (Dershewitz, 1975). If evidence can be accepted that such treatment at least prevents symptomatic urinary tract infection and possibly averts hospitalization, then neglect of the indications of urinalysis abnormalities is serious. Also, few would deny that finding proteinuria is worth immediate investigation. In this study, the physicians examined their own charts and admitted responsibility for the omissions, claiming that their patients were at serious health risk until a followup study was conducted.

Quality assurance implications confirm the value of a strategy of assessing outcomes and deductively identifying processes linked to deficient findings. The main problem, which is just as urgent today as it was at the time of the study, relates to the lack of physician motivation to follow unexpected abnormal routine screening results so as to improve the management they are providing to patients.

In this study, few questions were raised by the physicians involved as to the importance of the findings, especially in relation to possible urinary tract infections or other renal pathology. However, repeated effort to stimulate the individual physician to improve his or her performance in this regard failed. What is noteworthy, however, is the fact that when these physicians achieved little improvement individually, they acted jointly and established an administrative mechanism for tackling the problem. In this case, they arranged to have laboratory personnel follow all abnormal urinalyses with repeat tests, including bacterial cultures if smears revealed bacteria. If abnormalities were confirmed, especially in terms of existing bacterial infection, the attending physicians were notified so as to take appropriate

Table 9.11.   Health care assessment results in a study of abnormal urinalyses

Provider Characteristics	Patient and Sample Characteristics	Diagnostic Outcomes[a] (as percent in each category)			Sample Size (n) and Completion Rate (percent)	
		Obs	MAS		n	%
Study 1a Facility 1						
Community hospital in midwestern city. 114 physicians	Working and some middle class patients. Retrospective random sampling of laboratory test report file for 5 nonconsecutive months for unexpected abnormal urinalysis results[b]	(n = 164) Lack of minimum adequate response	83 ***	0	164	100

[a]Diagnostic outcomes measured in terms of physician response to abnormal test results.

[b]$\geq$ 1+ proteinuria and/or $\geq$ 5 white and/or red blood cells per high power field.

***P < 0.001

action regarding treatment. In this way, the inadequate response rate was probably significantly reduced. Unfortunately, there has been no followup study to assess the results after the introduction of this change.

Electrocardiograms

Topic. Two clinics jointly conducted a study of outcomes related to the provision of electrocardiograms. The providers were mainly primary care general practitioners and internists on the staff of two adjacent HMOs, and the patients were of working and middle class background from a western metropolitan city. In this study, both diagnostic and therapeutic outcomes were assessed.

Design. A retrospective consecutive sampling was conducted to identify patients possibly requiring an electrocardiogram, defined as all patients between 30 and 65 years of age seen at the clinic in a two-year period preceding the study. The total patient record file (approximately 5,500 charts) of both clinics provided the sample frame.

The assessment measure was a chart review form and an augmented patient health status questionnaire including the electrocardiogram indications shown in Table 9.12. A tabulation of positive indications for each patient was reviewed by a study team physician and checked as to whether the patient seemed to require an EKG. This list was compared to a separate tabulation indicating those patients having had an EKG as reported in their medical record. Patients requiring but not receiving this test were labeled "diagnostic false negatives," and those receiving but not requiring this test were labeled "diagnostic false positives."

Assessment standards were generated by the assessment study team, which consisted of members of the clinic staffs. By consensus, a maximum acceptable rate of false negatives and false positives was developed for diagnostic outcomes, and a frequency distribution of 100 hypothetical patients across the six level health scale was developed to indicate maximum acceptable group disability.

Results. Review of charts for 2,603 walk-in patients for the two year study period revealed 1,602 at risk—i.e., between ages 30 and 65. All charts were assessed, with 78 percent yielding sufficient data. Of the 95 patients found to require an EKG, 77 were subsequently lo-

Table 9.12.   Electrocardiogram indications in a study of patients thirty to sixty-five years of age

Study 44		
Disease/Syndromes	*Symptoms/Signs*	*Test Results*
Hypertension	Chest pain	Abnormal chest x-ray
Obesity	Shortness of breath	(arteriosclerotic findings or cardiac
Previous heart disease	Heavy smoking ($\geqslant$ 2 pkg/day)	enlargement)
Present heart disease	Syncope	Previous abnormal
Diabetes mellitus	Arrhythmia	EKG
Hypercholesterolemia	Sudden blindness	
Fluid in chest	Dizziness	
Calcified heart valves	Fundoscopic changes	
	Tachycardia/bradycardia	
	Pedal edema	

cated and interviewed, for an 81 percent response rate in relation to therapeutic outcomes.

Diagnostic outcome assessment revealed a 27 percent false negative rate, indicating serious underutilization of this test compared to standards (1 percent). The 7 percent unnecessary EKGs—i.e., false positives—was well within standards (15 percent). The health outcomes for the patients interviewed were also within standards (Table 9.13).

Implications.   The clinical implications of this study are that of those requiring an EKG by team standards, one in four did not receive this test, a finding clearly requiring inquiry to identify the determinants of this deficient outcome. One wonders whether this finding, in conjunction with the low percentage of false positives, reflects the often mentioned inclination of HMO physicians to be ultraconservative on medical care provided. Electrocardiogram utilization would seem a risky area in which to be conservative.

Although the topic selection thus proved accurate in identifying a serious care deficiency, it failed to stimulate any followup action by staff to effect improvement. While EKGs rarely indicate early cardiac disease, the screening criteria established by the staff (see Table 9.12) would certainly yield a high proportion of patients with late stage disease, based on age alone. Perhaps this study group was dubious about the health benefit possible even if the EKG revealed acute

Table 9.13. Health care assessment results in a study of adults at risk of requiring electrocardiograms

Provider Characteristics	Patient and Sample Characteristics	Diagnostic Outcomes[a] (as percent in each category)		Therapeutic Outcomes (as percent at each level)		Sample Size (n) and Completion Rate (percent)			
		Obs	MAS	Obs	MAS	Diagnostic n	%	Therapeutic n	%
Study 44 Facility 15 and 16									
HMO in western metropolis. 17 physicians	Working and middle class adults. Retrospective sampling of patient record file for consecutive patients seen within 2 years and considered at risk (30–65 years of age); one to three year followup of those found to require EKG	(n = 95) False negatives	27*** 1	(n = 77) Asymptomatic, normal risk	62	60	1602	78	95	81
		(n = 74) False positives	7 15	Asymptomatic, high risk	4	2				
				Symptomatic	28	30				
				Restricted	5	6				
				Dependent	1	2				
				Dead	0	0				

[a]Determined by independent chart review matching EKG indications with reported EKGs.

***P < 0.001

abnormalities, again a risky assumption. More likely, however, this study is an example of the general apathy of most physician groups toward focused quality assurance activity, an attitude that could pose a serious motivational barrier to subsequent action. Much additional research will be required to identify the behavioral determinants of this problem.

The finding of patient health status as well within standards could reflect invalid standards or, more likely, that the health status scale is not sufficiently sensitive to reveal a health problem of high risk of future impairment as opposed to one of immediate disability. The followup interval of eighteen months used in this study would probably not be sufficiently long for many patients to develop acute cardiac problems, and an interval of five years would probably indicate much more health dysfunction in this group. The question of how much difference early EKG screening can make in terms of patient health is an issue that requires considerably more inquiry, however; until this is resolved, it will be difficult to generate much concern about physician neglect of this test for general screening purposes.

Intravenous Pyelograms

Topic.   The same two clinics jointly conducted an outcome study for use of intravenous pyelograms (IVPs). The providers were primary care physicians in two adjacent HMO clinics, and the patients were from middle and working class backgrounds in a western metropolis. Both diagnostic and therapeutic outcomes were assessed.

Design.   Retrospective consecutive sampling of all 6,000 charts for patients seen in a thirty-month period was the basis of the diagnostic study, and a random sample of patients who had received an intravenous pyelogram was chosen for the fifteen-month followup assessment of health and disability status.

The assessment measure was a chart review form and a patient interview questionnaire. The study team established independent criteria for determining when an intravenous pyelogram should have been considered by the attending physician to be indicated—i.e., the list in Table 9.14, where Items 1, 2, or 8 required at least one other indication. Findings were tabulated and reviewed, and diagnostic outcomes were classified as false negatives if the patient had IVP indications by the above criteria but no record of this test was reported in the chart and as false positives if the patient had an IVP but chart evidence did not indicate this test to have been required.

Table 9.14. **Intravenous pyelogram indications in a study of diagnostic outcomes**[a]

Study 45	
1. Unexplained urinary tract infection	8. Unexplained hematuria
2. Recurrent urinary tract infection	9. Unexplained flank pain
3. Pyelonephritis	10. Kidney stones
4. Urine sediment (> 8 WBC or 1-2 RBC per high power field)	11. Hypertension
5. Benign prostatic hypertrophy in patients > 55 years	12. Family history of congenital kidney disease
6. Unexplained pelvic or abdominal mass	13. Any evidence of uretral obstruction
7. Renal failure BUN > 20 TP > 8 Albumin > 5	14. Trauma to kidneys

[a]Items 1, 2, or 8 in conjunction with at least one other indication.

Assessment standards were set by the staff physicians on the study team indicating the maximum acceptable false negative and false positive rates for IVP utilization, and the distribution of 100 hypothetical patients across the six levels of the health status scale indicated the maximum acceptable overall disability for the total group to be interviewed fifteen months after having received an IVP.

Results. All 6,000 charts were reviewed to identify patients either requiring or receiving an IVP. A random sample of 100 patients out of the 110 who had received an IVP was contacted. A health status interview was completed for 84, yielding a response rate of 84 percent.

The assessment findings are summarized in Table 9.16, which shows that both the proportion of those requiring but not receiving an IVP (35 percent) and of those receiving but not requiring this test (30 percent) far exceeded maximum acceptable standards. Table 9.15 delineates the frequency distribution of indications for an IVP in the false negative group. Therapeutic outcome assessment of the respondent group who had received an IVP was well within maximum acceptable standards for overall health status.

Implications. From a clinical point of view, the deficiencies in diagnostic outcomes related to this test were marked. With regard to the percentage of false negatives, one can only speculate about the extent of health benefit lost due to neglect of this radiological test. Earlier diagnosis of operable lesions producing obstructions, of

Table 9.15.   Intravenous pyelogram indications in forty-two patients not receiving this test

Study 45	
IVP Indications	Number of Patients
Unexplained flank pain	28
Recurrent urinary tract infection	17
Abnormal urinalysis	11
Pyelonephritis	9
Hypertension	7
Unexplained hematuria	4
Benign prostatic hypertrophy	2
Renal failure	1
Kidney stones	1

[a] Any one patient may have had more than one indication.

congenital deformities, and perhaps of tumors might have been possible. However, the degree of probability of identifying such pathology might be questionable. On the other hand, the number of those who received an IVP where it was not required raises questions regarding both the study criteria and the criteria applied by the physicians who ordered this procedure. Here, one must weigh the probability of unnecessary health risk (allergic reaction to the dye), discomfort, and expense caused to the 30 percent classified as false positives (i.e., patients receiving but not requiring an intravenous pyelogram).

The results of this study did not stimulate further inquiry. Again, one must ask whether this was a conscious decision based on a low probability of clinical benefit (in which case the initial selection of this topic must be questioned) or whether some additional mechanism is necessary to bring such findings to the attention of the HMO administration and physicians. This apathy is rather common in regard to much present quality assurance activity.

The lack of significant health deficiency in the group that had received an IVP is not surprising. In the light of diagnostic outcomes, nearly a third of this group did not require the test in the first place, and since most renal disease identified by this test is of a chronic nature, additional health impairment would not be likely to be evident in the fifteen month followup period. More convincingly, however, it can be argued that maximum acceptable standards were set unreasonably high, such that moderate disability in the group would not seem unusual. Accepting a 10 percent case fatality rate in the

Table 9.16. Health care assessment results in a study of patients receiving or requiring intravenous pyelograms

Provider Characteristics	Patient and Sample Characteristics	Diagnostic Outcomes[a] (as percent in each category)		Therapeutic Outcomes (as percent at each level)			Sample Size (n) and Completion Rate (percent)			
		Obs	MAS		Obs	MAS	Diagnostic n	%	Therapeutic n	%
Study 45 Facility 15 and 16										
HMOs in a western metropolis. 17 physicians	Working and middle class patients. Retrospective sampling of 6000 consecutive charts (30 months) for patients with intravenous pyelograms indicated or received; 15 month followup of random sample of patients given IVP	(n = 119) False negatives 35***	8	(n = 84)			6000	100b	100	84
		(n = 110) False positives 30***	10	Asymptomatic, normal risk	37	5				
				Asymptomatic, high risk	23	6				
				Symptomatic	26	50				
				Restricted	13	22				
				Dependent	1	7				
				Dead	0	10				

[a] False negatives defined as patients not receiving IVP despite one or more indications and false positives as patients receiving IVP in the absence of sufficient indications (see Table 9.14).
[b] Assumed; actual denominator not stated.
***P < 0.001

fifteen months after IVP administration seems overly pessimistic, as does accepting 29 percent away from major life activity or worse. At the very least, the study findings should have stimulated these physicians to reconsider the prognostic judgment implied by their outcome standards in regard to the population of their patients currently receiving IVPs.

PRENATAL SCREENING

Topic
One hospital elected to study outcomes with regard to uncomplicated term deliveries in the hospital. The providers were a group of board certified specialists in obstetrics and gynecology; the patients were working and middle class females in a midwestern city. Both diagnostic and therapeutic outcomes of medical care were to be assessed in terms of prenatal screening and of prenatal and peri-delivery complications and mortality.

Design
Diagnostic outcomes in terms of the provision of prenatal screening for urinary tract infections, diabetes mellitus, anemia, and cervical carcinoma were to be assessed. The study team drew a retrospective consecutive sample of 100 women who had delivered at the hospital in a three month period. The assessment measure consisted of a chart review to identify evidence of screening for bacteriuria, elevated two hour postprandial blood sugar, hemoglobin of less than 10 grams or between 10 and 12 grams, and cervical cancer.

Also, a two year retrospective consecutive sample of in-hospital normal obstetrical deliveries was checked to study therapeutic outcomes. The assessment measure consisted of a tabulation of prenatal complications and of maternal and perinatal mortality. Finally, an independent screening of a retrospective consecutive sample of medical records for close to 600 patients was conducted to check for prevalence of preventable complications associated with delivery. The assessment measure was a simple tabulation of any of the following problems:

- Anemia (degree not stated)
- Hemorrhage and shock
- Puerperal infections
- Pyelonephritis
- Puerperal psychosis
- Toxemia

Maximum acceptable standards for the incidence of these complications were set by the study team based on available literature data. Standards were also established indicating the acceptable percentage for the omission of prenatal screening tests as well as for maternal and perinatal mortality and prenatal and peridelivery complications, although no consensus on standards was reached for high risk urinary tract infections or hemoglobin levels of between 10–12 gm/100cc.

Results
Table 9.17 tabulates the results of the prenatal screening assessment. In terms of adequacy of routine prenatal screening, a check of 81 consecutive charts revealed deficient diagnostic screening outcomes in relation to the detection of urinary tract infections, diabetes mellitus, and cervical carcinoma. Only hemoglobin screening proved acceptable. In terms of therapeutic outcomes, the prevalence of prenatal complications, of maternal and perinatal mortality, and of peridelivery complications was within acceptable standards.

Implications
The clinical implications of this study are dubious. Although screening outcomes were deficient for urinary tract infections and diabetes mellitus, the measured prevalence of these complications did not indicate serious resulting problems. Indeed, there currently may not be consensus among investigators that such screening is efficacious in facilitating prevention of subsequent complications. Assessment findings in terms of maternal and perinatal mortality indicate clearly acceptable results in this facility.

The quality assurance implications of this study are more interesting if somewhat discouraging. While the study team was unable to generate standards for judging the acceptable prevalence of urinary tract infection of high risk status or for hemoglobin levels of 10–12 gm/100 cc blood in their patients, they went ahead and measured such cases anyway. These two instances illustrate the futility of expending effort on assessment measurements when standards cannot be satisfactorily established.

Another major problem of the study relates to the documentation of the multiple different samples of patients studied. It is presently not possible to determine valid results from such a variety of different sample sizes, nor can the completion rates for their assessment be established. Such information is vital, however, for interpreting results. If meticulous attention is paid to such tasks during an evaluation, the value of the overall effort, particularly in terms of generalizability of results, can be greatly enhanced. However, there was a

Table 9.17.   Health care assessment results in a study of uncomplicated term deliveries

Provider Characteristics	Patient and Sample Characteristics	Prenatal Screening Outcomes[a] (as percent in each category)		Complications and Mortality[b] (as percent in each category)	
		Obs	MAS		Obs	MAS
Study 6 Facility 1						
Community hospital and fee for service group clinic in midwestern city. 114 physicians	Working and middle class females. Retrospective consecutive sampling (3 months) of in-hospital term deliveries for minimum required prenatal screening; 2 year retrospective consecutive sampling of all in-hospital normal deliveries for mortality; and consecutive sampling of medical records of term deliveries for prenatal and peridelivery complications			*Prenatal complications* (n = 407)		
				Urinary tract infections (n = 179)	8	5
		(n = 81)		Anemia	8	11
		Urinalysis 94***	2.5	*Peridelivery complications* (n = 569)		
		Postprandial blood sugar 99***	7.5	Anemia	5	10
		Hemoglobin 7	2.5	Shock and hemorrhage	1	4
		Cervical smears 51***	5	Infections, puerperal	1	10
				Pyelonephritis	1	10
				Puerperal psychosis	0.2	0.25
				Toxemia	1	2.5
				Mortality		
				Maternal[c] (n = 3613)	2.8	3.6
				Perinatal[d] (n = 3605)	32	34

[a] Measured as percentage of patients for whom required screening procedures were omitted.
[b] Assessment numerators only available for this study; sample denominators were not stated except for prenatal screening, where it is 100.
[c] Per 10,000 deliveries
[d] Per 10,000 live births.
***P < 0.001

clear lack of enthusiasm by the obstetrical staff for assessing out-comes on this topic at all. Their collective judgment was that this would not be a fruitful area in terms of identifying educational needs and achieving improvement. Their assumptions were thus tested in this study and found valid. A subsequent grant was later obtained by the author to test the reliability and validity of just such aggregate judgments (Horn and Williamson, 1977). Results to date strongly support the premise that medical care providers, at least collectively, have a fairly accurate intuitive sense as to performance strengths and weaknesses.

REFERENCES

Dershewitz, R. 1975. Urinary tract infection—prevention, recurrence and significance. Conclusions from the literature. Baltimore: Johns Hopkins School of Hygiene and Public Health (processed).

Horn, S.D., and Williamson, J.W. 1977. Statistical methods for reliability and validity testing: an application to nominal group judgments in health care. *Med Care* 15:922-28.

Karger, S. 1959. *Documenta Geigy: Scientific Tables.* 5th ed. New York: Geigy.

McKeown, T., ed. 1968. *Screening in Medical Care—Reviewing the Evidence.* London: Oxford University Press/Nuffield Provincial Hospitals Trust.

University Group Diabetes Program. 1970. A study of the effects of hypoglycemic agents on vascular complications in patients with adult-onset diabetes, pt. 1: Design, methods and baseline results; pt. 2: Mortality results. *Diabetes* 19 (Suppl. 2): 747-87, 787-830.

Williamson, J.W; Alexander, M.; and Miller, G.E. 1967. Continuing education and patient care research—physician response to screening test results. *JAMA* 201:938-42.

Williamson, J.W.; Horn, S.D.; Choi, T.; and White, P.E. 1977. Evaluating an outcome-based quality assurance system. Final Project Report, Grant 5-R01-HS01590, National Center for Health Services Research, Department of Health, Education and Welfare, Baltimore: Johns Hopkins School of Hygiene and Public Health (processed).

Chapter 10

Health Accounting Outcome Studies: Psychiatry, Family Planning, and Satisfaction with Care

This chapter reports outcome assessment studies on relatively unconventional topics. Seven psychiatric outcome assessment studies will be described, three relating to general psychiatric care of specified population groups, two to drug abuse by adolescents and adults, one to depression, and one to aspects of adolescent sexuality. Furthermore, family planning outcome assessment will be presented, related primarily to contraceptive management, as well as an exploratory study of patient satisfaction with care received.

PSYCHIATRY

General Psychiatric Care

Topic. The health problems selected in three psychiatric outcome studies were a conglomerate of mental and emotional problems faced by defined populations. The providers were faculty members of the department of psychiatry in a prestigious medical school working in a university sponsored health maintenance organization in two studies and psychiatrists on the staff of a large multispecialty group in one study. In Study 16, the population was restricted to children and adolescents below age 18 from a middle class suburb in the eastern United States, presenting with a psychiatric complaint as their major problem. Study 17 related to adults between ages 25 and 50 from the same community, also presenting with a psychiatric complaint as their major problem. Study 26 focused on all patients receiving initial hospital or clinic care for a psychiatric problem during a four month period in a large rural catchment area. The focus was on the perceived resolution of problems and satisfaction with care (Study 16); on health outcomes related to specific psychiatric symptoms (Study 17); and on general health status (Study 26).

Design. In the psychiatric study of children and adolescents (Study 16), patients were retrospectively sampled to include patients to age 18 presenting with an initial psychiatric complaint as their major problem in the HMO clinic during a three year period. The followup period ranged from two months to three years. A computer list of patient visits provided the sampling frame for the final sample of 118 patients. Assessment was based on a three page questionnaire mailed out to the parents of all children and adolescents in the sample and on a separate questionnaire mailed to all adolescents above age 13. The parent questionnaire asked for the source of referral to the HMO clinic psychiatry service; the primary reason for referral (see Table 10.1); the intensity of their child's problems, feelings, or sensations at time of referral and at followup; the length of time from referral to being seen in the clinic; the number of and time intervals between visits for this problem; the reason for terminating care; and satisfaction with care. The adolescent questionnaire was essentially the same and allowed comparison of parent and adolescent perception of the problem and the outcome of care. Followup reminder letters were sent to those not responding.

Assessment standards were established by group consensus in terms of both health status and patient satisfaction outcomes. The study team indicated that maximum acceptable standards would be met even if as many as 70 percent of the problems were not resolved and if as much as 30 percent of all parents and of the adolescent patients were dissatisfied with care received.

In the adult psychiatric study (Study 17), patients age 25 to 50 were retrospectively sampled from computerized lists of clinic patients seen during the past two years. All medical charts were reviewed for patients having a psychiatric problem as the major complaint (marital problems were included). The followup period ranged from ten to fourteen months after treatment. Patients having terminated treatment at least five months previously made up the sample of 102 persons who were sent a one page questionnaire asking which of eleven categories of symptoms (see Table 10.1) best described their problem; which of four levels of intensity applied to their feeling about each symptom ("not at all distressed" through "extremely distressed"); and where, in the patient's perception,

Table 10.1. Child and adult symptom categories used in a psychiatric outcome assessment questionnaire

Studies 16 and 17	
Child Categories[a]	*Adult Categories*
Anxiety symptoms (fear, worry, nightmares, etc.)	Thoughts of ending your life
	Feeling of being trapped or caught
Withdrawal behavior (daydreaming, shyness, etc.)	Worrying or stewing about things
	Feeling hopeless about the future
School problems	Feeling easily annoyed or irritated
Aggression (temper tantrums, disobedience, cruelty, etc.)	Temper outbursts you could not control
Antisocial behavior (such as delinquency)	
Difficulty with peer relations	Feeling inferior to others
Bodily symptoms	Having to avoid certain things, places, or activities out of fear
Habit formation problems (bedwetting, eating, sleeping, etc.)	Feeling tense or keyed up
Sexual difficulties	Nervousness or shakiness inside
Hyperactivity	Feeling depressed
Depression	
Self-destructive behavior	

[a]Primary reason for referral.

effectiveness or success of treatment received in terms of symptom relief would be rated on a four point scale ranging from "not at all" (unsuccessful) through "very much" (successful).

Assessment standards were developed by team consensus methods projecting both how patients would be likely to respond under present care and how they might respond under ideal conditions of care, which assumed the following patient care improvements to have been accomplished:

- An increase in number and diversity of providers to eliminate the long waiting lists for appointments;
- An increase in referral service; and
- Provision of a day care hospital with both inpatient and outpatient facilities available.

Ideal standards were stated in terms of the respective percentage distributions of the total patient group across all items in the questionnaire and were to be compared to expected and observed percentage distributions.

In Study 26, all inpatients and outpatients ages 18 through 45 who were seen for the first time at the clinic psychiatric center in a four month study period were sampled, with the exception of those mentally retarded (IQ less than 80), patients with chronic brain syndrome, epileptics, and patients with gross physical illness or handicaps such as blindness, metastatic carcinoma, or active tuberculosis.

Each patient in the 100-person sample was followed for three to eight months, for an average of six months, and was contacted by phone or mail to complete a health status questionnaire indicating total functional impairment on a modified six point health and disability scale, as well as a series of ten questions focusing on the status of the major psychiatric complaints and further details as to occupational and social functioning. Finally, a question regarding satisfaction with care received was included.

Standards were provided by study team consensus regarding the frequency distribution of the total group over the six level health scale that represented maximum acceptable total group disability (see Chapter 6).

Results. In Study 16, parents of 64 of 118 children and adolescents in the sample and 22 of the 53 adolescents in the sample responded, for a 54 and 42 percent response rate, respectively; in only 16 instances were both parent and adolescent questionnaires returned. In Study 17, 69 of 102 patients in the sample responded, for a 68 percent response rate; and in Study 26, 87 out of 100 patients, for an 87 percent response rate (see Table 10.2).

In Study 16, the low response rates seriously limit interpretation of the percentage of patients whose problems were controlled, which was well within provider standards, as was the percentage of those who claimed to be satisfied with the care received. It is of interest, though, that in those instances (16) where questionnaires from both parents and adolescents were obtained, the adolescent group claimed to be markedly less improved and less satisfied with the care received than observed by their parents.

In Study 17, the response rate (68 percent) was appreciably better, though probably insufficient for generalizability. Overall, group impairment in terms of intensity of symptoms was well within standards at the end of the followup interval. Looking at individual items in terms of ideal standards, the findings shown in Table 10.3 are of interest.

For the two most serious symptoms (thoughts of ending your life, feeling hopeless about the future), findings seemed within ideal standards and were certainly better than expected. The 22 percent

Table 10.2.   Health care assessment results in three studies of mental and emotional problems in psychiatric patients

Provider Characteristics	Patient and Sample Characteristics	Therapeutic Outcomes[a] (as percent at each level)	Obs	MAS	Sample Size (n) and Completion Rate (percent) n	%
Study 16 Facility 5						
University prepaid HMO in an eastern metropolitan region. 45 physicians	Middle class children and adolescents. Retrospective sampling of computerized patient record (3 years) for consecutive patients < 18 years with initial psychiatric problems; 2 months to 3 year followup	Problems not resolved				
		Parent claim (n = 64)	52	70	118	54
		Adolescent claim (n = 22)	32	70	53	42
		Dissatisfied with care				
		Parent (n = 64)	30	30	118	54
		Adolescent (n = 22)	40	30	53	42
Study 17 Facility 5			Obs	MAS	n	%
University prepaid HMO in an eastern metropolitan region. 45 physicians	Middle class adults. Retrospective sampling of computerized patient record (2 years) for consecutive patients aged 25–50 years with psychiatric problems as major complaint having terminated treatment at least 5 months prior to sampling; 10–14 month followup	Aggregated levels of distress for 11 symptoms				
		(n = 69)			102	68
		Extremely	3	9		
		Quite a bit	12	13		
		A little	28	40		
		Not at all	57	38		
Study 26 Facility 9			Obs***	MAS	n	%
Private fee for service clinic in a rural midwestern town. 115 physicians	Working and middle class adults. Prospective sampling of consecutive new admissions ages 18–45 to psychiatric center; 3–8 month followup	(n = 87)			100	87
		Asymptomatic	24	40		
		Symptomatic	52	47		
		Restricted	18	11		
		Dependent	5	1		
		Dead	1	1		

[a]Measured in terms of perceived problem resolution and satisfaction with care received (Study 16) and of patient distress at specific problems (Study 17).

Note: In Tables 10.2–10.9, the abbreviations Obs and MAS denote, respectively, observed results and maximum acceptable standards. See Chapter 7 for methods used to determine statistical significance.

***P < 0.001

Table 10.3. Observed, expected, and ideal outcomes for symptom categories in a group of sixty-nine adult psychiatric patients

| | Study 17 | | |
| | *Outcome (percent)* | | |
Symptom Category	*Observed*	*Expected*	*Ideal*
Thoughts of ending your life	1	14	6
Feeling of being trapped or caught	22	25	13
Worrying or stewing about things	41	33	20
Feeling hopeless about the future	14	22	10
Feeling easily annoyed or irritated	23	30	22
Temper outbursts you could not control	9	20	12
Feeling inferior to others	9	26	14
Having to avoid certain things, places, or activities out of fear	10	20	10
Feeling tense or keyed up	36	30	19
Nervousness or shakiness inside	29	29	20

claiming a feeling of being trapped or caught, while worse than ideal standards, was close to the expected proportion. On the other hand, the distress from worrying, anxiety, and tension was far worse (by nearly a factor of two) than ideal standards and significantly worse than expected.

In Study 26, overall group impairment was significantly worse than maximum acceptable impairment standards (see Table 10.2). The major determinants of this outcome seemed to be the high proportion of patients still dependent on others for self-care activities and/or restricted from their major life activity.

Implications. At least as based on staff standards, child and adolescent psychiatric care seems to have been adequate in terms of problem control. Adult psychiatric care seemed far less adequate, especially in dealing with worry, tension, and anxiety. This area is now receiving much popular attention in terms of such treatment methods as biofeedback and meditation. Perhaps further clinical attention should be addressed to the management of patient life stress management, which may well be causing serious emotional distress as well as physical disability through such mechanisms as hypertension and its related complications, e.g., strokes and coronary insufficiency.

The quality assurance implications of these studies are obvious. In both HMO studies, the university psychiatric staff refused to apply the standard health scale to measure group disability on the grounds that this scale was inappropriate. One would think that overall quality of life, which the six level scale crudely approximates, should be central to psychiatric concern. The psychiatrists in the rural clinic had no difficulty with the scale and applied it meaningfully, identifying serious problems in care outcomes. The university psychiatrists also had difficulty in distinguishing "expected findings" from assessment standards in terms of maximum acceptable group disability. To approximate the latter concept, they identified specific structural improvements essential to improved health outcomes of their patients. One wonders if these staff attitudes are typical of other prestigious university faculties, who sometimes seem to assume that whatever results they are achieving must be ideal, regardless of evidence to the contrary.

This attitude does not facilitate assessment by objective methods. Is a standard of 70 percent of child psychiatric problems not relieved by treatment within three years indeed acceptable? Further inquiry into the team's prognostic judgment would seem indicated to provide more substantial evidence for such pessimistic standards. Finally, the surprisingly poor response rates achieved highlight the problem faced in many quality assurance projects conducted by university faculties, compared to the high response achieved with similar patient populations in studies conducted by nonacademic personnel. Such results would indicate that low priority is given to quality assurance investigations in academic settings.

Drug and Tranquilizer Abuse

Topic. Two urban HMO clinics elected to study the abuse of narcotics and of tranquilizers and antidepressants. The provider group in both clinics consisted of family practitioners, pediatricians, and internists. In the narcotics study, many of the staff were affiliated with a nearby university medical school. In the tranquilizer–antidepressant study, the staff were employees of a large for profit corporate health care group. The patient population in the narcotics study (Study 51) consisted of all enrollees in a university-affiliated HMO adolescent program in a poverty section of an eastern metropolis. The program provided for regular monthly visits for supportive therapy, drug education, and counseling by a specialist; enrollment in mental health service programs; and/or hospitalization if necessary. The patient population in the tranquilizer-antidepressant study (Study 41) consisted of all enrollees ages 18 through 55 seen in a suburban HMO in a poverty section of a large western city.

The assessment focus in both studies was health outcomes; in the tranquilizer–antidepressant study, diagnostic and projected economic outcomes were also studied with regard to overutilization of the following brand name drugs: Elavil, Equanil, Librium, Mellaril, Miltown, Meprobamate, Stelazine, Thorazine, Triavil, and Valium.

Design. In Study 51, medical records of all enrollees in the adolescent program were reviewed for evidence of usage of narcotics. Out of 1,829 enrollees, a sample of 128 was chosen by random selection. Each was classified in one of four categories:

- No evidence of usage,
- High risk though no immediate evidence of usage,
- Less than one instance of usage per week, or
- More than one instance of usage per week.

A one year followup was conducted from time of enrollment in the program to determine the health status of each adolescent in the sample. Assessment standards were developed by staff consensus. A frequency distribution of all patients in each of the four drug abuse categories was developed across five levels of the standard health scale, modified to account for relevant outcomes, as shown in Table 10.4.

In the tranquilizer–antidepressant study (Study 41), 5,200 medical charts for consecutive walk-in patients were examined for patients aged 18 to 55 and seen in a five month period. This yielded 1,842 patients, of whom 239 had received prescriptions for the tranquilizers and antidepressants listed above. The use of these pharmaceuticals was considered unnecessary if

- The patient had been given more than two refills for an acute self-limited health problem; or
- The patient had no recorded emotional or musculoskeletal disorder justifying such medication.

A one in two sample of all patients was followed one month after the last clinic visit; patients were interviewed by phone or in person, using the standard six level health scale questionnaire to determine health outcomes.

Assessment standards were set by team consensus, establishing the maximum acceptable percentage of patients receiving unnecessary prescriptions (labeled false positive drug indications). A frequency distribution across all six levels of the standard health scale was determined to indicate maximum acceptable group disability. Finally, potential economic gains and losses were projected, based on the assumption that all unnecessary prescriptions could be eliminated.

Results. In Study 51, out of a sample of 128 adolescents in the narcotics program, 90 (71 percent) responded to the health questionnaire that was administered approximately one year following enrollment in the program (Table 10.4). Assessment revealed the health outcomes for the enrollees in the adolescent program to be within standards. The majority seemed to be off narcotics by their own statement and according to available records. Only 5 had been classified as regular users, with 27 being at high risk of use.

In the tranquilizer–antidepressant study (Study 41), 21 percent of the sample were found to have received unnecessary prescriptions. This finding was within maximum acceptable standards. Among the 98 (82 percent) responding on followup, group disability was likewise well within acceptable standards. In terms of economic outcomes, it was estimated that the unnecessary drugs cost the HMO $1,390 (1972 dollars); this was compared to the more than $11,000 total required for each of these patients to have seen a psychiatrist for thirty minutes in lieu of the prescription.

Implications. While the care provided in both studies seems quite effective in terms of the standards established, before and after data would have been valuable, together with compliance information, to provide evidence for the attribution of care provided to outcomes measured. Also, is there no health risk for the one in five receiving unnecessary prescriptions?

On the other hand, quality assurance implications of these studies indicate either poor judgment in selecting topics with little appreciable health improvement potential, or invalid evaluation results. The data, especially the followup response rate in Study 41, seem to indicate rather well implemented studies. It is a matter of conjecture whether health outcome standards were realistic in the absence of a literature survey indicating efficacy of the health care involved and/or the natural history of untreated patients.

Depression

Topic. Another university sponsored HMO clinic studied the outcomes of depression as reflected by scores on the Minnesota Multi-

Table 10.4.   Health care assessment results in two studies of drug and tranquilizer use in adolescents and adults

Provider Characteristics	Patient and Sample Characteristics	Diagnostic Outcomes[a] (as percent in each category)		Therapeutic Outcomes[b] (as percent at each level)		Sample Size (n) and Completion Rate (percent)			
		Obs	MAS	Obs	MAS	Diagnostic n	%	Therapeutic n	%
Study 51 Facility 21									
University affiliated prepaid HMO in eastern metropolis. 3 physicians	Poverty class adolescents. Retrospective random sampling of program enrollees (1,829) classified into four drug use categories on the basis of chart review[c]; 1 year followup from time of enrollment							128	71
				(n = 90)					
				In school or on the job 71	42				
				In school or on the job, with significant absenteeism or poor performance 14					
				Out of school, on parole or probation, off the job > 3 days/week	42				
				In jail or hospitalized 13	15				
				Dead 2	1				
				0	0				

Study 41 Facility 14		Obs	MAS		Obs	MAS n	%	n	%
Corporate prepaid HMO in western metropolis. 13 physicians	Poverty class adults. Retrospective sampling of medical charts for consecutive walk-in patients aged 18–55 years seen in 5 month period; 1 month followup of one in two sample of those given tranquilizer or antidepressant prescriptions					1842	100	120	82
	(n = 239) False positives	21	20						
				(n = 98)					
				Asymptomatic, normal risk	33	8			
				Asymptomatic, high risk	2	10			
				Symptomatic	4	7			
				Restricted	58	72			
				Dependent	3	3			
				Dead	0	0			

[a] Defined as prescribed use of tranquilizers or antidepressants in the absence of positive indications in patient's medical chart.
[b] In Study 51, scale reflected relevant outcomes rather than overall health and disability.
[c] Only five enrollees were classified as regular users and twenty-seven as at high risk of use.

phasic Personality Inventory (MMPI). The providers were HMO staff on a university medical school faculty providing primary medical care to the HMO enrollees. Most were psychiatrists, internists, and pediatricians serving a population of enrollees who were predominantly black (86 percent), young (68 percent below age twenty), and female (86 percent). The assessment focus was on both diagnostic and therapeutic outcomes of care.

Design. A random sample of 250 patients age 14 and above was selected from the sample frame of 2,095 program enrollees. Diagnostic outcomes were established by review of the HMO medical records and diagnostic register for evidence that the staff were screening or managing any of the patients in the sample for depressive illness, the results being compared to those from a questionnaire mailed to each patient in the sample and consisting of the 60 true-false items of the MMPI depression scale. All patients responding to the original questionnaire were contacted by phone and given a standard health and functional disability questionnaire, expanded to include more specific MMPI items related to depression. A uniform strategy of callbacks was to be applied to improve the response rate for those not answering the telephone on the first call.

Outcome standards were established by the clinic quality assurance board consisting of the medical director; the directors of psychiatry, pediatrics, and nursing; and the administrator. Using formal consensus methods, the maximum acceptable rate of missed diagnoses (false negatives) and the percentage distribution of patients on the six level health scale were identified.

Results. Of the 250 MMPI questionnaires mailed out, only 96 (36 percent) were returned. Attempts to contact the 96 by phone succeeded for only 62 patients, for a final response rate of 63 percent of the sample contacted and 25 percent of the original group studied. Diagnostic outcomes in terms of false negatives far exceeded maximum acceptable standards, as did health outcomes (Table 10.5), where the proportion dependent on others for activities of daily living was eight times that considered an acceptable outcome.

Implications. Since the low response rates do not permit generalization, clinical implications are confined to the group studied. For this group, there seems to be a serious lack of recognition, in the medical records, of patients with a potentially disabling problem that is amenable to efficacious clinical intervention. The severity

Table 10.5.   Health care assessment results in a study of depression in adolescents and adults

Provider Characteristics	Patient and Sample Characteristics	Diagnostic Outcomes[a] (as percent in each category)		Therapeutic Outcomes (as percent at each level)			Sample Size (n) and Completion Rate (percent)			
		Obs	MAS		Obs***	MAS	Diagnostic n	%	Therapeutic n	%
Study 56 Facility 22										
University prepaid HMO in an eastern metropolis. 17 physicians	Poverty class adolescents and adults. Retrospective random sampling of enrollees above 14 years; follow-up of enrollees responding to depression questionnaire	(n = 96) False negatives 85***27		(n = 62)			250	36	96	63
				Asymptomatic, normal risk	17	7				
				Asymptomatic, high risk	8	37				
				Symptomatic	25	41				
				Restricted	25	11				
				Dependent	25	3				
				Dead	0	1				

[a]Measured as depression screening not provided by clinic staff although indicated by positive findings on Minnesota Multiphasic Personality Inventory depression scale.

***P < 0.001

of group functional disability seems especially distressing. If 25 percent of an essentially young age group are dependent on others for self-care activities, considerable clinical investigation would seem to be required, and the potential for improved diagnostic procedures and care should be explored.

There are two important quality assurance implications in this study. First, the low response rate to the initial questionnaire seriously limits the meaning of this study. All clinics, especially inner city HMOs, face high turnover rates and administrative record deficiencies. To assure high response rates, a multimodal outreach approach is essential. The success of Brook's sampling of both poverty and working class populations in Baltimore (Brook, 1974) illustrates how response rates in excess of 90 percent can be achieved. A combination of mailouts, telephone calls, and personal contacts in the clinic or at the patient's home are both feasible and practicable if resources are allocated for such a strategy. A rule of thumb is that at least 50 percent of survey resources should be expended on the last 33 percent in the sample who do not respond to initial contact.

Second, this study raises the question of the validity of pencil and paper tests for screening depressed patients. These instruments may be considered to be sensitive to mood and to reflect transient feelings rather than severe illness. However, since data of sufficient reliability and validity are available to support instruments such as the MMPI, it is doubtful whether this is a serious question (Welch and Dahlstrom, 1956). Sophisticated investigators would probably not question this instrument as such, but might challenge the use of one of its scales separately from, and out of the context of, the whole 450–500 question "long version." In the face of practical constraints, the value of such scales seems to outweigh their limitations, however. This is especially true if they are used primarily for screening and if it is assumed that there will be more adequate psychiatric diagnostic evaluation of patients receiving high scores on such scales.

Adolescent Sexuality

Topic.   One of the urban clinics in the health accounting project also elected to study adolescent sexual activity in a group of poverty class, inner city teenagers enrolled in an adolescent health program. The providers were the staff of a university affiliated HMO that was one of several clinics in a large health insurance plan of an eastern metropolis. Overall evidence of sexual activity was to be assessed in this prospective, longitudinal study.

Design. A sample of approximately 125 adolescents was randomly selected for a prospective longitudinal study from the pool of 1,829 adolescents enrolled in the health plan. Baseline data and one year followup data were obtained. The assessment measure, a modified health scale as shown in Table 10.6, was applied before and after a one year special adolescent counseling program for inner city teenagers.

Standards were developed by methods eliciting clinic staff consensus and indicating overall maximum acceptable group disability in terms of a percentage distribution of the group across all levels of the health scale.

Results. Complete baseline data were obtained for the total sample of 124 adolescents, and followup data for 87, for a 70 percent completion rate. Table 10.6 shows results for only the 87 for whom complete initial and final data are available. Accepting the ordinality (rank order levels) of the modified health scale that this study team designed, the overall status of this patient group was well within standards at the time of the first assessment. Of greater interest was the increased "impairment" noted one year after counseling. Sexual activity was the reason for the shift from 16 to 32 percent into the "at risk" category. If, as the scale implies, active sexuality in adolescents is undesirable and associated with increased health risks, the counseling is not working or might possibly be encouraging sexual permissiveness. Then again, perhaps it was simply one year's maturation of the group that was responsible, independently of the program.

Implications. It is difficult to establish the clinical relevance of these results, since they are so dependent upon one's value system. Some would hold that efforts with regard to adolescent sexuality might be more productive if applied to contraceptive counseling. Certainly some supportive evidence of the extent of implied health risks for this age group would help. The incidence of venereal disease and unwanted pregnancy would certainly be of greater clinical relevance and amenable to study, if merely by a brief literature review.

The quality assurance implications of this study relate to both topic selection and health scale development. It is not clear why and to what extent this study team considered adolescent sexuality a serious health risk. It is difficult to document the extent to which psychological and social impairments are causally related to early sexual activity. Some might argue that sexual abstinence might indicate greater future health risk. Even if early sexual activity is the

Table 10.6.   Health care assessment results in a study of adolescent sexuality

Provider Characteristics	Patient and Sample Characteristics	Therapeutic Outcomes[a] (as percent at each level)	Obs	MAS	Sample Size (n) and Completion Rate (percent) n	%
Study 52 Facility 21						
University affiliated inner city HMO in eastern metropolis. 3 physicians	Poverty class adolescents. Prospective random sampling of 1,829 health plan enrollees; longitudinal followup over 1 year counseling program	*First Assessment* (n = 87)			124	70
		Healthy—sexually inactive, in school or at work	71	38		
		At risk—sexually active, in school or at work	16	57		
		Symptomatic—sexually active, in school or at work	8	2		
		Dependent—sexually active, dropped out of school or work	5	3		
		Dead	0	0		
		Second Assessment (n = 87)			124	70
		Healthy—sexually inactive, in school or at work	57	38		
		At risk—sexually active, in school or at work	32	57		
		Symptomatic—sexually active, in school or at work	6	2		
		Dependent—sexually active, dropped out of school or work	5	3		
		Dead	0	0		

[a]Measured as level of sexual activity at beginning and end of followup period.

greater risk, however, how effective are counseling programs in reducing such risk? Value clarification is essential in such care programs.

This problem illustrates the difficulties that arise when topics are selected without careful consideration of the specific disabilities involved and of the epidemiology of these disabilities, as well as the hazards of not considering the efficacy of available treatment modalities. Why assess health impairment if it is uncertain whether health care makes a difference? Such information, for example from longitudinal studies or controlled clinical trials, must be available before assessment studies can be planned or their results interpreted.

The modification of the standard health scale to better suit the population and health problems involved was important, however. Levels 4 (restricted) and 5 (dependent) were combined in this study due to the reduced probability that many would be at those levels. Defining active sexuality as Level 2 (at risk) was interesting but controversial, as discussed above, since it implied a putative health impairment only.

FAMILY PLANNING

Topic

Unwanted pregnancy and contraceptive management were selected by one clinic for quality assurance study. The providers were primary care physicians on the staff of a university affiliated HMO; patients consisted of poverty class, inner city females, 12 to 45 years of age. Both diagnostic and therapeutic outcomes were assessed, diagnostic outcomes being defined in terms of the proportion of sexually active women who did not desire pregnancy but were not receiving any contraceptive management (false negatives), and conversely, of the proportion of women who desired pregnancy but were receiving, or had received, unwanted contraceptive management (false positives).

Design

Sampling was conducted on the basis of medical charts for female enrollees who were age 12 to 45 years, had been in for initial history taking and physical examination, and had a telephone. Of approximately 2,000 enrollees, charts were available for sampling for only 1,135 patients. Of this group, 266 were age 12 to 45, and of these, 236 had a telephone. A random sample of 129 charts was drawn from the 236 eligible. Of the 129, 44 proved ineligible either because the telephone listed had been disconnected (30), or the woman proved not to be in the required age range (12), or had not been seen or was disenrolled (2). The final sample thus contained 85 women of a total 236 eligible.

The assessment measure consisted of a chart review form and of a patient interview questionnaire designed to elicit the standard information for classifying the patient at one of the six levels of the health scale. Questions were included to identify those sexually active (at risk of pregnancy), those who did or did not desire pregnancy, and those presently receiving or not receiving some form of contraceptive management. Contraceptive management included any of the following: birth control pill, intrauterine device, diaphragm, foam, condom, hysterectomy, rhythm method, douche, withdrawal, vasectomy of spouse, or tubal ligation.

Assessment standards were defined by the study team in terms of diagnostic outcomes, i.e., maximum acceptable proportion of false negatives or false positives, and of therapeutic outcomes, i.e., the distribution of 100 hypothetical patients on the six level health scale to represent maximum acceptable group disability.

Results

Assessment of diagnostic outcomes revealed serious deficiency in terms of patients at risk for an unwanted pregnancy, i.e., not receiving contraceptive management when indicated (needed *and* wanted), as shown in Table 10.7. Only one patient desired pregnancy and had an unwanted hysterectomy, an overall finding (5 percent) within standards.

Additionally, review of the 266 charts for females aged 12 to 45 revealed 13 abortions during the study period. There was reason to believe this number to be a low approximation of total abortions received. Therapeutic outcome assessment, however, was within maximum acceptable group disability standards, with 81 percent of the sample responding.

In order to provide a validation check, the team was also asked to estimate the diagnostic outcomes that were likely to be found on measurement. Such estimates must be distinguished from maximum acceptable standards, which involve a value judgment, as opposed to outcome estimates, which are predictions of measured findings. A comparison of the diagnostic outcomes predicted by the study team with measured findings is shown in Table 10.8, which seems to support the predictive judgment of the staff involved in this study.

Implications

The clinical implications of this study are that nearly half of an inner city female sample desiring contraceptive management did not

Table 10.7. Health care assessment results in a study of contraceptive management of adolescent and adult females

Provider Characteristics	Patient and Sample Characteristics	Diagnostic Outcomes[a] (as percent in each category)		Therapeutic Outcomes (as percent at each level)		Sample Size (n) and Completion Rate (percent)			
						Diagnostic		Therapeutic	
		Obs	MAS	Obs	MAS	n	%	n	%
Study 54 Facility 22									
University sponsored HMO in eastern metropolis. 17 physicians	Poverty class females. Retrospective/prospective sampling of 1,135 available medical charts for enrollees 12–45 years of age having had initial examination and available for telephone interview; random sample of those eligible	(n = 33) False negatives 42*** (n = 20) False positives 5	5 5	(n = 69) Asymptomatic, normal and high risk 84 Symptomatic 4 Restricted 6 Dependent 6 Dead 0	82 12 4 1 1	85	81	85	81

[a]False negatives defined as at risk of unwanted pregnancy but receiving no contraceptive management and false positives as receiving contraceptive management when not indicated or desired.

***P < 0.001

Table 10.8. Estimated as compared to measured diagnostic outcomes and to maximum acceptable standards in a group of women screened for contraceptive management

	Outcome (percent)		
	Predicted	Measured	MAS
Not receiving contraceptive management although at risk	44	42	5
Receiving contraceptive management when not required	7.5	5	5

in fact receive it. Further inquiry is needed to determine what type of patient or physician education is required to change this outcome.

Quality assurance implications are of special importance in this study. The limitation of the survey to women who had a telephone eliminated nearly one in four otherwise eligible women. Mailout questionnaires or house calls have proven quite successful in many other studies and might have been used more effectively here. Many recent surveys of inner city populations have had better than 80 percent response rates by a multimethod approach and some extra effort (Brook, 1974). In addition, the fact that the investigators in the present study depended upon medical records to provide the sample frame resulted in the loss of another 43 percent of the total enrolled population. Quality assurance samples in HMOs have a notable sampling advantage in enrollment rosters. Ideally, these should be used to provide the universe from which samples are drawn for studies such as this one. Admittedly, this involves outreach surveys. But in view of the proven success of health accountants completing such tasks, clinics should be encouraged to plan more comprehensive sampling strategies.

The estimates of outcomes made by this clinic staff add to the mounting evidence that staff judgment regarding predicted outcome deficiencies is often borne out by actual findings. It is now recommended that health accounting study teams routinely make such estimates in the planning stage of assessment studies. If outcome predictions from present performance are close to maximum acceptable standards (which they were not in this study), the team should think twice before planning to move ahead on an outcome assessment for that topic.

SATISFACTION WITH CARE

Topic

One clinic conducted an outcome assessment study of patient satisfaction with health care. The provider group was the staff of a fee for service and prepaid multispecialty group practice located in a rural midwestern town. The patient population in this case was the student body of a small private college. The outcome topic was satisfaction with the care received at this clinic.

Design

The student directory for the college was sampled retrospectively to obtain an 8 percent sample, which was to be contacted for a personal interview approximately two weeks prior to the end of the school year. The assessment measure was an interview form requesting specific reactions to clinic visits as well as overall reactions to health care provided. Students were considered ineligible if they had not visited the clinic within a year. Permission was obtained from each student interviewed to review his chart. The chart review form covered the number of visits and the type of each visit, whether problem oriented (illness related) or routine (immunizations, physicals, etc.).

Analysis consisted of a simple correlation of all visits mentioned in the personal interview to the chart review data for that visit. Tabulation was by college year, as well as by type of visit and degree of satisfaction. In this exploratory study, assessment standards were implicit in that any dissatisfaction expressed was to be considered grounds for investigation so as to gain insight into the students' feelings about the health care provided by the clinic.

Results

The sample consisted of 200 students, of whom 31 had not been to the clinic in the past year; 6 refused to complete the interview or would not give permission for a review of their medical record. Of the 163 for whom an interview was completed, charts could not be located for 2. Complete information was thus compiled for 161, for a 95 percent completion rate (Table 10.9). According to the medical records, a total of 615 visits had been made to the clinic by the respondents, of which 149 were not mentioned in the interview (122 problem oriented visits and 27 routine visits). Table 10.9 shows the study findings as a distribution of respondents over four satisfaction levels.

Table 10.9.   Health care assessment results in a study of satisfaction with care

Provider Characteristics	Patient and Sample Characteristics	Therapeutic Outcomes (as percent at each level)		Sample Size (n) and Completion Rate (percent)	
			Obs	MAS[a]	
				n	%
Study 23 Facility 10					
Fee for service and prepaid clinic in a rural mid-western town. 16 physicians	College students. Retrospective sampling of student directory for students with clinic visits within 1 year. Followup questionnaire on satisfaction with health care	(n = 161)		169	95
		Totally satisfied	39		
		Generally satisfied	51		
		Partially dissatisfied	10		
		Very dissatisfied	0		

[a]Maximum acceptable standards not set in this exploratory study.

Implications

These patient satisfaction outcomes are difficult to interpret in the absence of both standards and data regarding health outcomes. How many dissatisfied patients would be required to indicate further inquiry? The usual predominance of satisfaction by patients reporting on their physicians was noted, although 39 students complained of an inadequate physical examination. As patients generally tend to express satisfaction to providers of care on whom they may depend for medical help, serious underreporting often precludes valid measurements.

Most providers of health care are interested in patient satisfaction assessments, if for no other reason than the wish to avoid malpractice suits. However, satisfactory methods for measuring this type of outcome are still at a very early stage of development. Close attention to reliability-validity studies on this topic is strongly recommended to those who would allocate quality assurance resources for this purpose.

SUMMARY

Analysis of the outcome assessment projects implemented in the first ten years of health accounting (1963-1973) revealed important clinical and methodological findings. In addition to confirming the feasibility of conducting numerous prospective and retrospective assessments of diagnostic and therapeutic outcomes by clinic teams inexperienced in survey research, the analysis permitted determination of the statistical significance of the findings despite the wide range of sample sizes and survey methods. Assessment methods and results across 56 quality assurance projects comprising a total of 87 studies, which extended from care for organic medical disease to psychiatric procedures and drug counseling, were presented in Chapters 8-10 in standard tables, showing individual sample sizes, completion rates, and assessment results. Individual project designs and findings were described on a comparable basis, the projects being grouped by health problem or medical care focus and discussed in terms of topic selection, study design, diagnostic and therapeutic results, and their implications as to both clinical aspects and quality assurance.

The reliability and validity of the health and functional ability scale applied in most of these projects clearly requires further study. As a crude initial screening instrument, it seems to have sufficient face and content validity, however, to warrant application until more definitive evaluation data are available.

REFERENCES

Brook, R. 1974. *Quality of Care Assessment—A Comparison of Five Methods of Peer Review*. Rockville, Md.: Department of Health, Education and Welfare, Publication No. (HRA) 74-3100.

Welch, G.S., and Dahlstrom, W.G. 1956. *Basic Readings on the MMPI in Psychology and Medicine*. Minneapolis: University of Minnesota Press.

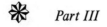 *Part III*

The Next Step

Chapter 11

The Implications of an Outcome Approach for the Development of Quality Assurance: Summary and Recommendations

Although quality assurance in the United States may well be the most advanced among comparable systems of health care (Reerink, 1977), little of its potential for improving population health and for a more efficient use of resources has been realized. Theoretical considerations relating to quality assurance concepts and requirements were discussed in Chapters 1-5, and several approaches were proposed with a view to developing more effective strategies for assessing and improving health care. Chief among these was an outcome approach to quality assurance that would widen the traditional understanding of health care outcomes and include measurable characteristics not only of health problem outcomes, but of provider, patient, and care interaction outcomes that are now often classified as health care processes. This redefinition of the outcome concept was used to develop the construct of achievable benefits of care, taking into consideration both provider and consumer values, so as to provide a basis for determining the extent to which achievable benefits of care are not being achieved.

The description and analysis, in Part II, of health accounting approaches and results has furnished initial evidence of the feasibility of translating these concepts into practical quality assurance activity in a variety of ambulatory and hospital care settings, where local characteristics of both patients and providers determined the selection of assessment topics and the setting of assessment standards. Important limitations of this overall experience must be recognized, however. As mentioned in Chapter 7, most health accounting projects to date have been carried out in multispecialty group clinics and associated hospitals. There has been no attempt to implement this approach in solo practice or in long-term care institutions such as nursing homes, although the needs in these settings for evaluation and improvement of care are pressing, as indicated in Chapter 4. Most providers have been primary care specialists such as internists and pediatricians as well as surgeons and psychiatrists. Few family or general practitioners have participated. Also, the projects encompassed only a small proportion of the practice of the participating facilities. Finally, institutional involvement with health accounting, or with any other system of quality assurance, was often limited. The traditional resistance to spending time and funds on assessment and improvement activities was observed in many places, though it proved a serious obstacle only in fee for service institutions. The voluntary contribution of time by professional staff concerned with productivity in terms of numbers of patients seen per day proved to be a not infrequent impediment. In spite of these limitations, the projects encompassed a wide range of populations, geographic locations, and health care personnel. The health accounting experience was enriched by the contributions of many, from lay members of boards of trustees to physicians, nurses, administrators and front desk employees.

On the basis of this experience several important planning requirements relating to scientific, technical, and management aspects can be formulated for future quality assurance systems:

- Quality assurance functions must be integrated into health care management operations instead of being relegated to a peripheral position.
- Problems significant for health improvement or cost reduction must be emphasized instead of those readily measurable (e.g., from existing medical record systems).
- Applicability to the entire range of health care, from ambulatory to hospital and long-term care facilities, and at individual and community levels, must be ensured, as well as adaptability to present quality assurance systems and functions.
- The reliability, validity, and cost effectiveness of assessment and improvement methods must be continually evaluated and the results applied to subsequent planning decisions.
- It will be necessary to develop a standard unit for quantifying health values and to formulate and test the instruments required for applying such units, so as to permit a more precise evaluation of improvement potential and cost effectiveness in the light of efficacy, effectiveness, and efficiency indicators.

- Organization of a national quality assurance research and development program is recommended to provide an institutional basis for coordinated planning and development of quality assurance methods, including the formulation of measurement instruments and the provision of training resources to facilitate the understanding of a wide variety of assessment and improvement modalities, and to permit the design of local quality assurance systems adapted to local needs and resources.

Such resources will be increasingly necessary if quality assurance efforts are to be directed to topics of realistic improvement potential at all levels of health care organization, whether in individual practice, in the community, or on a regional and national basis.

THE INTEGRATION OF QUALITY ASSURANCE FUNCTIONS INTO HEALTH CARE MANAGEMENT

Contemporary quality assurance is developing primarily in response to external pressures. For the most part, it is a peripheral function in health care institutions, and too often it has become a compliance operation generating reams of reports to satisfy accreditation and payment requirements but making very little difference to the health care delivered. A very limited segment of the professional staff in most institutions are in any way active in or even concerned with formal quality assurance. Very few medical audits result in substantial changes in care, so that current quality assurance is often seen as little more than a nuisance, leading mainly to improvements in medical record keeping. The Institute of Medicine of the National Academy of Sciences (1976) as well as the PSRO evaluation of the Office of Planning, Evaluation and Legislation (Health Services Administration, 1977) have documented similar findings in national evaluations of quality assurance activity, indicating that both current assessment and continuing education mechanisms appear to have limited effect in terms of patient health improvement or reduced costs.

It is the author's opinion that substantial improvement in health care outcomes is unlikely as long as major emphasis is on outside incentives and negative sanctions. Without question, some control will have to be exercised in this way, and some mechanism may be necessary to enforce compliance where all else has failed. What is more important to realize, however, is that the majority of health care providers are conscientious, responsible men and women who are constrained largely by present conditions of practice and by organizational and financial mechanisms that place major emphasis on care process and structure and that reward providers for what is done rather than for beneficial outcomes achieved. To be effective, future quality assurance systems will have to depend upon providers seeing beyond the borders of traditional medical care responsibilities and utilizing a much broader armamentarium of interventions to combat a far wider range of problems than those posed by acute organic diseases or impairments. For instance, better communication and health education skills will probably facilitate greater improvements in care than learning about recent enzyme research. The motivation to improve health outcomes should stimulate more innovative ways of looking at old problems and should lead to more meaningful relationships between providers, consumers, and others in the community. What is needed, among other things, is a more cooperative approach to assigning priorities for resource allocation that is related to achievable health outcomes.

Emphasis should shift from obsession with chemical nostrums for every ill to a more holistic approach based on encouraging both the well and the sick to assume greater responsibility for their own health care. The application of even crude measures of cost effectiveness in the allocation of health care resources might help check the trend to exploit every recent development in medical technology, at vast expense to the total population, to obtain diagnostic information that is far beyond what present therapeutic capability can utilize. How can such approaches to quantifying health care cost effectiveness be implemented? In the following, the development of relative and absolute indicators of performance on the basis of standard health value units is proposed, as well as a coordinated research and development program that can develop, test, and demonstrate means of educating both health care personnel and consumers of care in the principles of estimating those health and economic benefits of care that are in fact achievable.

QUANTIFYING THE BENEFITS OF CARE

To achieve tangible progess, it will be necessary, first, to define and develop a standard health value unit so that benefits and disbenefits of care can be quantified, projected health outcomes can be directly related to patient and provider values as well as to costs, and clinical and administrative decision makers can be educated to think in terms of cost effectiveness. If explicit, operational standard units of health value can be related to dollar costs for alternative management directions and improvement potential expressed in terms of achievable health benefits, health care personnel could be far more innovative in identifying explicit care objectives and in efficiently utilizing resources to achieve them. Such an approach might also allow physicians to see more clearly where they can best use their expertise and judgment, as well as those aspects of care where other health care personnel might take over a multitude of needed and critical tasks.

A Standard Unit for Measuring Health Value

The development of a standard, universally accepted unit measure of health value, comparable to monetary units that establish an indirect measure of value applicable to goods and services, is a critical need of an outcome approach to quality assurance. Such a standard unit of health value could help us to place the evaluation of care on a generally accepted basis of benefit desired as compared to benefit achieved, enabling a more uniform specification of health care objectives and a more meaningful evaluation of performance. Agreed statements of health achievement could be related to alternative care modes to facilitate clinical decision making; health units could be reflected in prognostic probability statements to indicate alternative risks of different management strategies, enabling the patient to assume his rightful role in making critical choices in an informed manner. The purchase of equipment or the construction of facilities could be assessed in terms of standard health value units and derived benefits and costs to be gained or foregone by alternative approaches. Management functions at all levels would be facilitated if a uniform basis for cost-effectiveness estimates in all sectors of the health industry were available (Goldschmidt, 1978).

The criteria for such a unit incorporate those described in Chapters 3 and 6 regarding the health status scale applied in health accounting:

- Applicability to all individuals regardless of how they are aggregated, and to all age levels;
- Adaptability to the entire spectrum of health, including both positive (higher levels of wellness) and negative (levels of disability or impairment) aspects;
- Independence of etiological factors and applicability regardless of the extent or complexity of physical, emotional, or social components;
- Independence as well of the natural history or treated prognosis of health problems; and
- Use of a ratio scale having an absolute zero (i.e., death).

The main problem in developing such a unit measure of health value is how to achieve a practical means for patients and providers, and for society as a whole, to express the relative value of differing health states in relation to their own personal and social life goals. Widespread use and application of such a unit will therefore require, in addition to the necessary research, an educational undertaking and social, ethical, and legal consensus. However, the health accounting experience has demonstrated, at least in terms of measurable health impairment, the need for a basic health value unit to facilitate evaluation of health care benefits and disbenefits and to achieve a final balance of overall accomplishment.

Development would have to occur in at least two basic stages: (1) conceptualization and definition of a unit for quantifying health value; and (2) phased development of instruments for eliciting and incorporating local population values. Clearly, establishing an acceptable measure reflecting the value of varying health states is a complex problem. Most current health scales relate to negative health only—that is, to disability or impairment—and do not encompass higher levels of wellness. It may thus be a practical necessity to start with the negative or impairment side of the health status scale. As more solid agreement is achieved on what should constitute levels of positive health, the other half of the scale could be added. The current development of "wellness medicine" by physicians such as John Travis illustrates some principles of positive health (Ardell, 1976), as does Maslow's hierarchy leading toward self-actualization (Maslow, 1968).

A unit of health value as recently applied to the estimation of achievable benefit in terms of reduced impairment (Williamson et al., 1977) incorporates health states and time. Here, health state represents the level of overall function limitation as measured on a six level scale. Time can be in any convenient unit from hours to decades, depending upon the application, and indicates how long the individual functions at each level of health limitation. In relation to both health states and time, however, each interval on the scale must be additive to all other intervals. To be additive, a health unit related to a patient being symptomatic but at full work activity must be considered equivalent to one related to a patient in a completely dependent status in a nursing home; a year of a child's life must be considered equivalent to a year of an adult's life.

To convert present ordinal health and time scales to interval or ratio scales, utility weights reflecting provider and consumer values must be developed and multiplied by, respectively, each health state and time unit. The development of specific weighting factors for both the time and the health state dimensions of the unit is required so that the value systems of the decison makers and the group to whom the decisions apply—the consumer or patient population receiving care—can be incorporated. The assumption here is that, though the concept of a health value unit might be universally acceptable, there is little likelihood of the formulation of a single set of utility weights for all subgroups of the population. Therefore, it will be necessary to develop practical means of eliciting and applying local value weights to local decisions. For aggregates of groups, averages or medians of the combined value weights for the aggregate would apply, so as to render the resulting units universally applicable across all subgroups for which individual group weights were incorporated.

Data Requirements for a Standard Health Value Measure

To obtain such standard health value weights, two questionnaires would be required to provide the needed data—health status over time, and health status and time (or age) utility values—on a sample basis. The measure of raw or unweighted health status would be based on a series of questions reflecting the length of time the patient spent at each level of the health state scale within the given time interval included in the unit. The remaining questionnaire would be a subjective probability instrument to reflect patient values in relation to the relative intervals on the health state scale and the time scale. These value weights could be considered constants for a given group in that they would have to be obtained relatively infrequently, assuming such values to remain stable. On the other hand, the health status scale measurements would have to be obtained periodically to measure expected change. Such instruments would have to be designed and pretested with random samples so as to provide both health status and value data applicable to a larger population constituting the sample frame.

At present, several crude health scales exist that might meet the requirements for health status data. The six level scale originally developed and modified for health accounting can be applied over the telephone, in person, or by mail (see Appendix A). A modified instrument developed by Gross (1977) yields a more precise measure of established reliability and construct validity. Other measures could be used, provided that their credibility and general acceptance were assured and that their reliability and validity could be shown.

What does not now exist is a practical, operational method for eliciting value weights to convert the ordinal health status scale to an interval or ratio scale. Progress has been made in this direction by some investigators (Kaplan, Bush and Berry, 1976). Also, practical procedures for eliciting value weights for each subgroup on a local basis remain to be developed.

Applying Health Value Units and
Measures to Quality Assurance

In Chapter 3, the derivation of indexes for quantifying efficacy and levels of care effectiveness and efficiency (see Figures 3.4–3.6) was demonstrated by means of an extrapolation from epidemiological data. To illustrate the feasibility of applying similar methods on the basis of standard benefit and cost units as suggested in the foregoing, it is assumed that a specific set of health care interventions can be related to outcomes of positive net value for individuals or populations and translated into specific benefit units, here expressed as health impairment unit years.

Application of a standard unit of health care value makes possible an essential differentiation between absolute and relative benefits that is usually obscured in evaluation systems. When stated as rates, indexes of value provide a relative measure of accomplishment only. Two care systems could thus achieve identical effectiveness ratings yet differ widely in absolute accomplishment. For purposes of discussion, let us assume two prepaid practices that are equal in terms of provider capability, patient populations, and health problems managed. Clinic A achieved aggregate benefits amounting to 8 lives saved out of 10 that would have been lost in the absence of quality assurance activity. Clinic B selected another set of topics, saving 80 lives out of 100 that might otherwise have been lost. Both clinics would have achieved identical effectiveness rates, namely, 80 percent in terms of relative benefit. Obviously, Clinic B accomplished ten times more when an absolute measure, here in terms of patient lives, is used. Clearly, absolute measures of quality assurance accomplishment are essential; relative measures, on the other hand, can provide meaningful indicators of potential and actual accomplishment.

An Illustration of Health Benefit Measures.   In five multispecialty clinics, outcome based medical care evaluation projects involved an aggregate of 7,069 patients and seven different health problems (Williamson et al., 1977). Health impairment was measured at the beginning of the year using an interval scale arbitrarily weighted by the author. For the 7,069 patients involved, an aggregate of 5,050 health impairment unit years were measured, of which 1,589 were considered remediable according to local staff judgment. This infor-

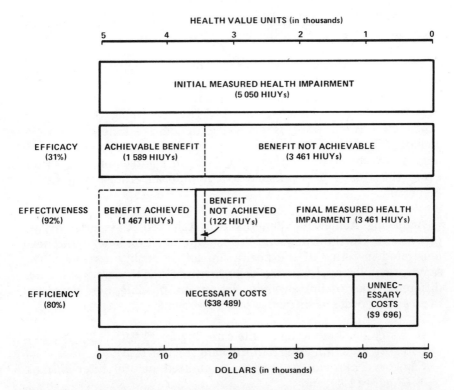

Figure 11.1. Assessing the outcomes of health care and quality assurance activity by means of efficacy, effectiveness, and efficiency indexes as based on aggregated measurements obtained in health accounting projects in five multi-specialty group clinics, 1974-1977. In this example, health value units are expressed in health impairment unit years (HIUYs), and the benefit achieved was measured after completion of the improvement stage. The extent of achievable benefit was based on local staff judgment of the limits of present health care potential and local resource capacity.

mation can be used to compute an adjusted quality assurance efficacy index of 31 percent, as shown in Figure 11.1. In other words, the clinic staff estimated that only one third of the measured health disability experienced by the above population could be eliminated in the following year with current technology and available resources. Of this improvement potential of 1,589 health impairment unit years, 1,467 were found to have been actually achieved at the end of the year, based on followup measurements. These findings can be used to compute an effectiveness index, which in this example would equal 92 percent, representing life years gained or years at lesser levels of impairment (see also Figure 3.3). In other words, over nine-tenths of the achievable benefit was actually achieved in these studies.

To illustrate this approach in terms of efficiency, Figure 11.1 also shows the total cost expanded on the benefit achieved, here expressed as the cost of the quality assurance activity in the five participating clinics. This cost was $48,185, of which $38,489 was expended on the projects achieving documented health benefit, including both direct costs (e.g., professional staff time) and 30 percent overhead rate costed out over an eighteen-month period. From these data, it is possible to compute an efficiency index of 80 percent.

Achieving Achievable Benefits Not Achieved: Categories of Improvement. In the foregoing, the use of evaluation indexes has been illustrated in terms of the health impact of quality assurance. The same principles apply to the assessment of health care itself. Four different types of improvement actions are possible, here described in ascending order of difficulty of achievement:

Category 1—Eliminating inutile care (Figure 11.2);
Category 2—Eliminating harmful care (Figure 11.3);
Category 3—Providing previously omitted helpful interventions (Figure 11.4); and
Category 4—Providing increased care capacity (Figure 11.5).

Category 1 (eliminating harmless but inutile care) results in improved efficiency but does not change effectiveness of health care. Examples of the potential for increased efficiency are the omission of low risk interventions such as drugs, certain minor surgical procedures, diagnostic methods, equipment, and other management modes for which there is no reasonable evidence of efficacy. Such procedures probably account for a substantial amount of present care expenditures. Also, innovations in patient management based on results reported from isolated case studies, on unreplicated research that has not been analyzed for validity, and on informal clinical experience in the day-to-day practice of medicine will have little likelihood of yielding substantial patient benefit. Eliminating such unproven or unnecessary care can significantly increase the overall efficiency index by reducing the total cost of care, as shown in Figure 11.2, with little likelihood of significant loss of benefit.

Category 2 (eliminating harmful care) also results in the improvement of efficiency; in addition, the effectiveness of care is enhanced.

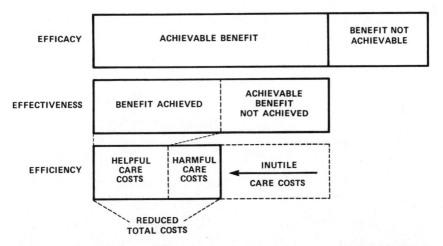

Figure 11.2. Eliminating inutile care to reduce total costs. The efficiency index rises, but the effectiveness index is unaffected.

Both efficiency and effectiveness can be increased by the identification and elimination of interventions considered as having a negative net value for a given problem—i.e. those that are harmful or unsafe, or of moderate to high risk with little or no health benefit (errors of commission), as shown in Figure 11.3. In practice, this implies elimination of contraindicated harmful interventions such as certain drugs, high risk diagnostic or surgical procedures, and destructive counseling or health education creating unnecessary anxiety or reduced compliance—e.g., the use of barbiturates in advanced emphysema, of chloramphenicol for nontyphoid infections, of tetracycline in children or of penicillin for common colds, or any unnecessary surgical or exploratory procedure, especially those requiring general anesthesia. It has been reported that more than 10 percent of surgical operations may be canceled if a second opinion is obtained (McCarthey and Widmer, 1974). Tonsillectomy rates may be three to four times higher, and hospitalization rates two to three times higher, in fee for service as compared to prepaid practice (Kristein, Arnold, and Wynder, 1977). Other examples are misguided complex interventions in a serious problem area where a high level of skill is required in terms of judgment, motorsensory functions, or interpersonal relations. The failure to recognize the limits of one's own abilities or those of staff and facilities may be very damaging at all levels, from technicians to tertiary specialists. There is evidence that subspecialists, when functioning outside their field of expertise, may be providing some of the least competent care (Payne et al., 1976;

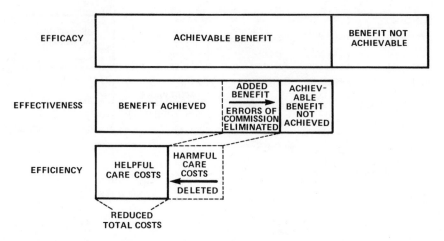

Figure 11.3. Eliminating harmful interventions (errors of commission) to increase benefit achieved and reduce total costs. Both the effectiveness and efficiency indexes rise.

Rhee, 1975). This is especially important in view of recent evidence from the National Ambulatory Medical Care Survey that secondary and tertiary specialists provide a considerable amount of primary care (Pushkin, 1977).

Category 3 (providing previously omitted efficacious care within reasonable cost constraints) will further increase effectiveness; this may be accompanied by an increase in care expenditure while efficiency remains constant, as shown in Figure 11.4. However, such errors of omission will only rarely consist of the neglect of dramatic breakthroughs in medical technology. More likely, they will consist in neglecting well-known and widely available health care interventions. Lack of an adequate medical history or physical examination probably results in far more missed diagnoses than failure to use new, sophisticated procedures such as computerized axial tomography. Lack of adequate care for the elderly or of rehabilitation for those suffering from chronic debilitating health problems, both physical and emotional, probably leads to far more unnecessary impairment than failure to prescribe miracle drugs. Ensuring awareness of available but neglected sources of efficacious health care and support is an achievable benefit that may well prevent or reduce considerable disability and discomfort, if not improve patient productivity and lifespan. Especially in metropolitan areas, many communities are developing directories of available health care resources, including financing, telephone counseling, rehabilitation, transportation, and child care services, that may not be widely known by the medical profession. These aspects, which are relatively new to the traditional field of medical care responsibilities, would appear to offer significant potential for improving the effectiveness of medical practice and health care.

Finally, Category 4 (increasing health care capacity) indicates that the potential for benefit from efficacious interventions can be realized to a greater degree by expanding local resources to more closely approximate ideal care conditions. As shown in Figure 11.5, this can result from additional expenditure augmenting the capability of a given provider or community. This requires a readjustment of provider values, however, and consequently a substantial upward adjustment of the local efficacy index may not be a realistic goal in many circumstances. Such improvements usually involve more costly and complex interventions, extensive systems changes, communitywide programs, or structural reorganization and thus lie outside the realm of institutional quality assurance activity. Perhaps the crucial quality assurance aspect in considering improvements in the efficacy index is a clarification of values and the setting of policy priorities. In deciding what level of benefit is achievable in the light of population needs, a compromise between breadth and depth of capabilities is necessary. The disbenefits involved in tertiary centers trying to expand their primary care capabilities beyond their interests or caring capabilities would seem to be similar to those likely to occur if

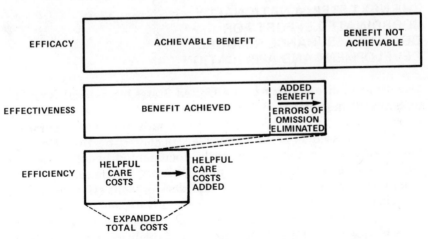

Figure 11.4. Utilizing previously neglected efficacious interventions (eliminating errors of omission) to increase benefit achieved. The effectiveness index rises but, while total costs rise, the efficiency index is not affected.

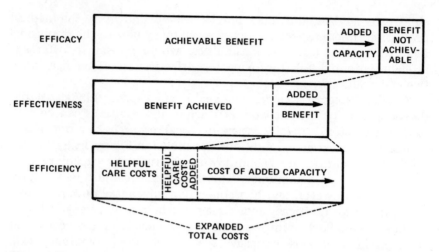

Figure 11.5. Augmenting provider or resource capacity to increase both efficacy and effectiveness of care. The efficacy index rises but, while total costs rise, the efficiency index is not affected. The effectiveness index is likewise unaffected.

primary care facilities expanded specialty and subspecialty resources beyond their interests and abilities. It is important to recognize these limits of both capability and capacity and of the range of resources that are reasonable in light of community health needs, provider interests, and consumer and provider values.

THE NEXT STEP: A NATIONALLY COORDINATED EFFORT FOR QUALITY ASSURANCE RESOURCE DEVELOPMENT AND APPLICATION

Quality assurance activity in the United States has expanded rapidly in terms of man hours and resource expenditures. Yet there is not much in the way of evidence that the results are commensurate to the effort. Providers are becoming disenchanted by the efforts required of them in the face of little documented benefit. To overcome the lack of direction that may well result from such conflicts, a nationally coordinated research and development effort appears to be called for, based on cooperation by private, public, and professional groups. To bring this about will require an imaginative approach. However, if a national program of quality assurance research and development could establish realistic goals and priorities, the present dominance of sectoral interests might yield to a more farsighted and broadly based policy.

At the present time, the main tasks of such a national program would seem to lie in applied research and development, information, and education, as well as demonstration and evaluation of practicable quality assurance systems and resources at all levels.

The research and development function should encompass study of more practical health scales, including methods for formulating and compiling value weights; of assessment instruments applicable to solo practice; and of educational resources for effecting organizational change. Quality assurance methods development should thus encompass clinical, administrative, and educational aspects of health care and should concentrate only on those methods and approaches that offer reasonable prospects of widespread application within specified and practical time and resource constraints.

An information compilation, validation, and indexing function is advocated to document the value of existing quality assurance strategies, interventions, and priorities in terms of health benefits and cost effectiveness. Quality assurance information requirements relating to observer error studies, the natural history of chronic and other disease processes, educational research, controlled trials and experimental studies related to clinical practice, as well as to specific studies of health care assessment and improvement and to reliability and validity documentation, can be more efficiently met if a system of reference coding for specific applications were to be provided.

The major educational function of a national program would be to fulfill training needs in terms of knowledge, skills, and attitudes for effective quality assurance at all levels of endeavor. Training of both medical professionals and nonprofessionals should be stressed. Personnel skilled in the design and implementation of outcome based quality assurance systems are needed, as are health educators who can implement validated improvement strategies in areas of clinical performance deficiencies and who can organize and train local personnel. The development and demonstration of patient self-care methods and of means of securing community organization of health programs are other educational needs. The basic assumption here is that a monolithic quality assurance system is neither the goal nor a prerequisite; instead, human and technical resources should be used to design and implement systems that can meet specific local needs in terms of patient populations, health problems, provider interests and facilities, and levels of performance.

The service function of such a program should lie in the provision of design and organization assistance and of evaluation and monitoring services to institutions where a continuing quality assurance program is not indicated for reasons of scope or funding. The availability of consultants who can provide information, analyze local needs, recommend suitable approaches, and coordinate ongoing quality assurance and continuing education activities would facilitate development in line with the requirements of local providers and communities. The essence of internal motivation is having a choice and not being unduly coerced, being stimulated by experience and trial applications as opposed to automatic enforcement mechanisms.

Where do we go from here? Increasing discontent with the direction of present quality assurance activities in this country is not encouraging. On the other hand, there is growing evidence that the need for fundamental change is slowly being recognized. If it is true that outcome based systems of quality assurance offer greater promise than those restricted to a review of medical records, then the methodological aspects of such systems, and the behavioral and organizational barriers to and incentives for their development and implementation must be better understood. It is hoped that the principles and results of the health accounting approach described in this book may contribute to a change in the present direction of assessment and improvement of care and prove helpful in developing cost effective, outcome based quality assurance systems.

REFERENCES

Ardell, D.B. 1976. *Meet John Travis, doctor of well-being. Prevention* 28(4): 62-68.

Goldschmidt, P.G. 1978. A model for measuring health status: application to the United States population. *J Comm Health* (in press)

Gross, R. 1977. Outcome measures of medical care: development and evaluation of a functional status measure for quality assurance. Master of Science thesis, Johns Hopkins University School of Hygiene and Public Health.

Health Services Administration, Office of Planning, Evaluation and Legislation. 1977. *PSRO: An Evaluation of the Professional Standards Review Organization.* Report Number OPEL 77-12. Rockville, Md.: Department of Health, Education and Welfare.

Institute of Medicine. 1976. *Assessing Quality in Health Care: An Evaluation.* Washington: National Academy of Sciences.

Kaplan, R.M.; Bush, J.W.; and Berry, C.C. 1976. Health status: types of validity and the index of well being. *Health Serv Res* 11:478-507.

Kristein, M.M.; Arnold, C.B.; and Wynder, E.L. 1977. Health economics and preventive care. *Science* 195:457-62.

Maslow, A.H. 1968. *Toward a Psychology of Being.* New York: Van Nostrand.

McCarthy, E.G., and Widmer, G.W. 1974. Effects of screening by consultants on recommended elective surgical procedures. *N Engl J Med* 291:1331-35.

Payne, B.C.; Lyons, T.F.; Dwarshins, L.; Kolton, M.; and Morris, W. 1976. *Quality of Medical Care: Evaluation and Improvement.* Health Services Monograph Series T40. Chicago: Hospital Research and Education Trust.

Puskin, D.S. 1977. Patterns of ambulatory medical care practice in the United States: an analysis of the national ambulatory medical care survey. Doctoral thesis, Johns Hopkins University School of Hygiene and Public Health.

Reerink, E. 1977. Personal communication.

Rhee, S.O. 1975. Relative influence of specialty status, organization of office care and organization of hospital care on the quality of medical care—a multivariate analysis. Doctoral thesis, University of Michigan.

Williamson, J.W.; Horn, S.D.; Choi, T.; and White, P.E. 1977. Evaluating an outcome-based quality assurance system. Final Project Report, Grant HS01590, National Center for Health Services Research, Department of Health, Education and Welfare. Baltimore: Johns Hopkins School of Hygiene and Public Health (processed).

✳ *Appendix A*

Health Status Questionnaire and Scoring Instructions

Appendix A reproduces the health status questionnaire developed for health accounting projects and used to determine the overall health status of patients for therapeutic outcome assessment studies. The questionnaire consists of two parts, the first establishing usual life activities and the second determining the respondent's overall health to approximate a measure of quality of life. The answers to questions about participation in usual activities, level of comfort, and dependency on others for self-care are scored as shown in the second section of this appendix, and the respondent is assigned to one of six health and functional levels on the following six level ordinal scale:

Level 1—Asymptomatic, normal risk
Level 2—Asymptomatic, high risk
Level 3—Symptomatic
Level 4—Restricted
Level 5—Dependent
Level 6—Dead

For details concerning questionnaire administration and aggregation and the assessment of questionnaire results, see Chapters 6-7.

HEALTH STATUS QUESTIONNAIRE FOR
INITIAL THERAPEUTIC ASSESSMENT

Name:_____   Date:_____

Address:_____   Sex:_____

Phone:_____   Age:_____

I would like to know about your present health and your level of activity in everyday living. This will give me some idea of how you are being helped by medical care and if improvement of the clinic's service is warranted. Would you please answer several questions?

1. At this time, what is your daily major life activity?

_____I am employed, full time (and not a student or housewife).
_____I am employed, part time (and not a student or housewife).
_____I am a student, not employed.
_____I am a student, employed part or full time.
_____I am temporarily unemployed.
_____I am a housewife, not employed.
_____I am a housewife, employed part time outside the home.
_____I am a housewife, employed full time outside the home.
_____I am retired and employed part time.
_____I am retired, not employed (and not permanently disabled).
_____I am permanently disabled.
_____I am temporarily disabled.

2. How would you rate your overall health and your ability to perform major life activity during the last four weeks?
   a. Are you able to participate in your major life activities, e.g., work, school, retirement, etc.?
   ___Always ___Most of the time ___Some of the time ___Never
   b. Do you have any medical problems?
   _____Yes _____No
   c. If yes,
      c.1. What are they?_____
      _____
      c.2. Which is the most serious problem?_____
      _____
      c.3. Does this problem cause you any pain or discomfort?
      _____Always _____Most of the time
      _____Some of the time _____Never

d. To what extent can you function in your major life activity?
__100% __75% __50% __25% __0%
e. Do you need help in caring for yourself in any of the following functions?
  e.1. Eating:
    __100% __75% __50% __25% __0%
  e.2. Dressing:
    __100% __75% __50% __25% __0%
  e.3. Bathing:
    __100% __75% __50% __25% __0%
  e.4. Going to the bathroom:
    __100% __75% __50% __25% __0%

GUIDELINES FOR SCORING AND INTERPRETING THE HEALTH STATUS QUESTIONNAIRE

General Remarks

The response to Question 1 is the basis for interpreting the responses to Questions 2.a and 2.d.

Questions 2.a and 2.d are crucial in determining the cutoff between Levels 3 and 4. A patient who can participate in his major activity always or most of the time and who functions 75–100 percent in this activity would be at Level 1, 2, or 3, depending on his reported medical problems and pain or discomfort. A patient who can participate in his major activity only some of the time or never and who functions less then 75 percent in this activity would be at Level 4 or 5, regardless of reported medical problems.

The distinction between Levels 4 and 5 is made by Question 2e, 1–4. A patient who needs help in any of the self-care functions 0–25 percent of the time would be classified at Level 4, while the patient who depends on others for help more than 25 percent of the time would be at Level 5.

Key to Scoring

Classify the patient at *Level 1, Asymptomatic, normal risk,* if his responses correspond to the following:
Q2.a.: Participation in major activity
    __X__Always (or) __X__Most of the time
Q2.b: Medical problems
    __X__No (or) __X__Yes
Q2.c.1 and 2: If yes, only self-limited problems or symptoms acceptable at this level e.g., mild and infrequent headaches, colds, sore muscles, fever, heartburn, etc.

Q2.d: Function in major activity
      _X_ 100% (or) _X_ 75%
Q.2.e.1, 2, 3, *and* 4: Need help with self-care functions
      _X_ 0%

Classify the patient at *Level 2, Asymptomatic, high risk,* according to the following responses:
Q2.a: Participation in major activity
      _X_ Always (or) _X_ Most of the time
Q2.b: Medical problems
      _X_ Yes
Q2.c.1 and 2: If yes, only chronic problems presently in remission (patient has had no symptoms in past month) are acceptable for this level, e.g., arthritis, hypertension, diabetes, etc. (The patient may say that he has the problem or may say that the doctor told him that he has the problem.)
Q2.c.3: Not applicable to Level 2 determination
Q2.d: Function in major activity
      _X_ 100% (or) _X_ 75%
Q2.e.1, 2, 3, *and* 4: Need help with self-care functions
      _X_ 0%

Classify the patient at *Level 3, Symptomatic,* according to the following:
Q2.a: Participation in major activity
      _X_ Always (or) _X_ Most of the time
Q2.b: Medical problems
      _X_ Yes
Q2.c.1 and 2: If yes, any problem acceptable except self-limited and chronic problems in remission (see Levels 1 and 2, Q2.c).
Q2.c.3: Pain or discomfort from medical problem
      _X_ Always (or) _X_ Most of the time (or)
      _X_ Some of the time
Q2.d: Function in major activity
      _X_ 100% (or) _X_ 75%
Q2.e.1–4: Not applicable for Level 3 determination

Classify the patient at *Level 4, Restricted,* according to the following:
Q2.a: Participation in major activity
      _X_ Some of the time (or) _X_ Never
Q2.b and c.1–3: Not applicable for Level 4 determination
Q2.d: Function in major activity
      _X_ 74–51% (or) _X_ 50% (or) _X_ 25% (or) _X_ 0%
Q2.e.1, 2, 3, *and* 4: Need help with self-care functions
      _X_ 25% (or) _X_ 0%

Classify the patient at *Level 5, Dependent,* according to the following:
Q2.a: Participation in major activity
<u>X</u> Some of the time (or) <u>X</u> Never
Q2.b and c: Not applicable for Level 5 determination
Q2.d: Function in major activity
<u>X</u> 25% (or) <u>X</u> 0%
Q2.e.1, 2, 3, *or* 4: Need help with self-care functions
<u>X</u> 100% (or) <u>X</u> 75% (or) <u>X</u> 50% (or) <u>X</u> 49–26%

Classify the patient at *Level 6, Dead,* according to the following: Patient's death confirmed by physician, medical record, or death certificate.
(*Note:* Cause of death should be determined and recorded for outcome analysis.)

Appendix B

The Costs of Health Accounting:
Selected Data on Manpower, Time,
and Financial Requirements

The following is a summary of quality assurance project costs in terms of manpower and time, providing an indication of health accounting funding requirements. Based on aggregated costs of several studies extrapolated to one health care facility assessing care for a subpopulation of approximately 6,000 patients a year, the figures cited here by way of illustration will undoubtedly vary among institutions; they are of a preliminary nature and include as well those costs incurred by the developmental aspects of the projects, such as training of staff, development of new resources, and reliability and validity testing. The data shown were compiled from seven health accounting projects conducted in six separate institutions subsequent to the projects reported in Chapters 8–10.

MANPOWER

The staff required in the implementation of a health accounting project includes the quality assurance coordinator, the health accountant, the priority team, and one study team for each project. The priority team selects topics for assessment of probable deficiencies and improvement potential for all quality assurance projects to be conducted in the facility. The quality assurance coordinator, usually a physician, organizes and trains the priority team and the individual study teams, coordinates the individual projects, and supervises the health accountant. The health accountant conducts the assessment activities, among them data collection and reporting of results. Each study team meets three or four times during each health accounting project to develop standards and measurement techniques, analyze initial assessment results, formulate improvement plans, and analyze reassessment results (see Chapter 5 for the composition and tasks of the study teams and Chapter 6 for details of the organizational structure, function, and stages of a health accounting project).

TIME

The health accountant is the only full-time project member. The quality assurance coordinator devotes 5 percent of his time to health accounting, and the priority team meets approximately five hours for quality assurance topic selection. The data shown in Table B.1 are based on two annual meetings, one for training and one in which all assessment topics were selected. This team usually includes seven members, of which at least four are physicians. Each of the study teams, usually consisting of five members (not all of them physicians), meets three to four times a year, their members contributing a total of approximately ten hours each per project.

COST

As shown in Table B.1, the direct costs for a health accounting project total $3,614 annually, on the assumption that six projects are conducted through five stages at one facility. This figure includes the annual salary of the health accountant, the cost of time devoted by the quality assurance coordinator, and overhead costs (computed at 30 percent of direct cost) such as data preparation and processing, and miscellaneous management and administrative costs. On the further assumption of six projects conducted at one facility and encompassing 6,060 patients in one year, direct per patient costs for the six quality assurance projects average $3.58.

Table B.1 shows the cost of priority and study team meetings as indirect costs, as these meetings take place during regular hours and in terms of time required are comparable to the range of staff meetings usually conducted at health care institutions. They thus do not involve overtime or other reimbursements for the health professionals involved. Considered as indirect health accounting costs, professional staff time assigned to priority team and study team meetings raises per project costs to a total of $4,810 or $4.76 per patient.

This total project cost is extremely close to results obtained by an independent cost analysis of health accounting conducted by two

Table B.1.   Illustration of manpower, time, and financial requirements of six health accounting projects (1977)

Manpower	Staff Time (percent)	Annual Cost ($)	
		Direct	Total[a]
Project Coordinator	5	2,600	
$52,000/yr = FTE/MD ($27.08/hr)			
Health Accountant	100	14,076	
Quality Assurance Teams			
Stage 1—Priority setting	5 hr/priority team member[b]		677
Stage 2—Initial outcome assessment	2.5 hr/study team member[c] (6 projects = 15 hr)		1,625
Stage 3—Definitive assessment and improvement planning	5 hr/study team member (6 projects = 30 hr)		3,250
Stage 4—Improvement action (no meetings)			
Stage 5—Reassessment	2.5 hr/study team member (6 projects = 15 hr)[d]		1,625
Subtotal		16,676	23,853
Overhead (as 30 percent of direct cost)		5,003	
Total		21,679	28,856
Cost per project		3,614	4,810
Cost per patient in sample population		3.58	4.76
Cost per total clinic population		0.12	0.16

[a] Including indirect cost.
[b] Priority team = 5 MD equivalents.
[c] Study team = 4 MD equivalents.
[d] Assumes additional tasks planned and implemented to achieve outcome standards.
Note: Costs based on actual data for seven projects completed through all five stages (1974–1977), extrapolated to 6 five stage projects conducted at one institution over one year and encompassing an aggregate study population of 6060 patients.

consultants from the Harvard University Center for Analysis of Health Practices (Shepard and Thompson, 1976).

REFERENCES

Shepard, D., and Thompson, M. 1976. A cost-effectiveness analysis of the health accounting project. Cambridge, Mass.: Center for the Analysis of Health Practices, Harvard School of Public Health (processed).

Index of Authors

Index of Subjects